From Band-Aids to Scalpels

Motherhood Experiences in/of Medicine

T0303635

Edited by
Rohini Bannerjee and Karim Mukhida

DEMETER

From Band-Aids to Scalpels

Motherhood Experiences in/of Medicine

Edited by Rohini Bannerjee and Karim Mukhida

Demeter Press
2546 10th Line
Bradford, Ontario
Canada, L3Z 3L3
Tel: 289-383-0134
Email: info@demeterpress.org
Website: www.demeterpress.org

Demeter Press logo based on the sculpture "Demeter" by Maria-Luise Bodirsky www.keramik-atelier.bodirsky.de

Printed and Bound in Canada

Cover image: Illustratrice Manu
Cover design and typesetting: Michelle Pirovich

Library and Archives Canada Cataloguing in Publication
Title: From band-aids to scalpels: motherhood experiences in/of medicine / edited by Rohini Bannerjee and Karim Mukhida.
Names: Bannerjee, Rohini, 1976- editor. | Mukhida, Karim, 1975- editor.
Description: Includes bibliographical references.
Identifiers: Canadiana 20200378074 | ISBN 9781772583328 (softcover)
Subjects: LCSH: Women in medicine. | LCSH: Women physicians.
| LCSH: Women medical students. | LCSH: Working mothers.
| LCSH: Mothers, Education.
Classification: LCC R692 .F76 2021 | DDC 610.85/2,Äîdc23

Contents

From Band-Aids to Scalpels: Motherhood Experiences in/ of Medicine

Rohini Bannerjee and Karim Mukhida

The intersectionality of medicine and motherhood is explored herein with fifteen distinct approaches. Academics, writers, thinkers, artists, scientists, health practitioners, and mothers from across three continents bring plume to paper on the topic of motherhood in/of medicine.

The topic of the call for papers for this issue was purposefully kept broad. We sought the perspectives of healthcare providers as mothers. As the medical profession has become more feminized (Levinson and Lurie; Potee, Gerber, and Ickovics; Walsh et al.), increasing attention has been paid to the experiences of physicians as mothers, which has included explorations of the stress that physician mothers experience during their pregnancies and their reentry to clinical work after parturition. Healthcare practitioners have reflected on the hidden costs physician mothers bear as they balance care for patients with care for family in a medical culture that can stigmatize and induce shame (Farid; Rangel et al.). It is not surprising to learn, then, that contemplations of motherhood by physicians also brings about contemplations about their career choice altogether (Huffmyer and Fahy). Thus, medicine as a culture needs to recognize the importance of caring for its physicians, just as it is expected that physicians care for others (Potee, Gerber, and Ickovics).

Additionally, we wanted to hear from mothers about their experiences interacting with the machinery and culture of medicine. What does the machinery of modern medicine look like when you are a mother whose child requires medical attention? How does a mother navigate through the medical system advocating for their own care or that of a loved one?

A set of chapters in this collection also looks at the topic of motherhood in/of medicine by examining the lived experiences of women of colour. Kimberly C. Harper's essay looks at Black maternal health by examining implicit bias within the context of patriarchal health workforces, whereas Alekhya Das's study explores the autonomy and agency of health-seeking women in the context of a slum neighbourhood in Delhi. Jeannette Wogaing meanwhile, looks at how female physicians in Cameroon experience and manage their own maternity in the context of a country that has high maternal mortality.

The role mothers play in the care of their children is also better understood in this collection. Catherine Ma's contribution discusses the need to build a collaborative approach that includes the mother when caring for paediatric patients. The beneficial but also potentially burdensome implications of such collaboration are explored in Celeste Orr and Amanda Watson's piece, which looks at mothers' unique involvement in their intersex children's so-called treatment.

Two contributions explore the theme of advocacy when it comes to creating community and a sense of belonging for mothers. Darryn Wellstead investigates how mothers use Facebook groups to talk and make decisions about health, and Hannah Rochelle Davidson argues for a stronger clinical recognition of postpartum depression in order to build further support for mothers.

The first-person narratives to this collection bring together a diverse array of lived experiences. Ariel Watson's provocative piece on the violation of informed consent asks readers to reevaluate the effects of obstetrical interventions on mothers. Anna Johnson speaks, via her performative anecdote, on the unique experience of mothers with chronic illnesses. The challenges of being both mother and physician are brought to life in the chapters by Arundhati Dhara, Ajantha Jayabarathan, and Sally Bird. Dhara's reflections illuminate the invisibility of the work she does both as a family physician and as a mother and asks readers to contemplate the emotional and physical burnout that physicians as mothers face when those roles are superimposed. Jayabarathan describes the juggling act of being the good doctor and the often absent mother while challenging expectations of what a balanced life might look like. Bird discusses the gender parity inequities faced as both a pregnant postgraduate trainee and a staff physician married to another physician.

What happens when the physician mother becomes ill? Sharon McCutcheon generously shares her powerful prose of resilience as her identity shifts from physician mother to neurosurgery patient. She helps readers better grasp the lack of support often endured by patients, especially those balancing their roles as mother and physician. Erin Northrup and Hannah Feiner write from the perspectives of children witnessing their physician mothers fight illness. In Northrup's case, she explores the gaps within the medical system with respect to supporting physicians who are mothers. In Feiner's piece, about her attempt to manager her medical career, mothering, and chemotherapy, the voice of her young daughter is heard throughout.

We thank the contributors to this issue for bringing together these experiences, stories, and studies of motherhood and its manifestations in/of medicine.

Works Cited

Farid, H. "Hidden Costs of Motherhood in Medicine." *Obstetrics and Gynecology*, vol. 134, 2019, pp. 1339-41.

Huffmyer, J. L., and B. G. Fahy. "Cracking the Motherhood and Medicine Code." *Anesthesia & Analgesia*, vol. 130, no. 5, 2020, pp. 1292-95.

Levinson, W., and N. Lurie. "When Most Doctors Are Women: What Lies Ahead?" *Annals of Internal Medicine*, vol. 141, no. 6, 2004, pp. 471-74.

Potee, R. A., A. J. Gerber, and J. R. Ickovics, "Medicine and Motherhood: Shifting Trends among Female Physicians from 1922 to 1999." *Academic Medicine*, vol. 74, no. 8, 1999, pp. 911-19.

Rangel, E. L., et al. "Perspectives of pregnancy and motherhood among general surgery residents: a qualitative analysis." *The American Journal of Surgery*, vol. 216, no. 4, 2018, pp. 754-59.

Walsh, A., et al. "Motherhood during Residency Training." *Canadian Family Physician*, vol. 51, no. 7, 2005, pp. 991-97.

Chapter 1

Implicit Bias, Visual Rhetoric, and Black Maternal Health: Understanding the Real Risk Factor

Kimberly C. Harper

Introduction

When a child is born, typically the birth announcement provides the weight, length, and sex followed by the cliché: "Mother and baby are doing fine." This sentiment rings true for many families; however, there are times when the mother is not fine. Television and movies romanticize giving birth with exaggerated scenarios of a woman's water breaking, a scared father delivering his child in a taxi, or a woman pushing during labour for a few minutes and then being handed her child as she laughs, cries, and chats with medical staff and family. As a society, we have been conditioned to see birth as a process that is free from complications rather than the life or death event that it is. Some have even called birth the closest a living person can come to death without dying due to the enormous amount of stress placed on the mother's vital organs. In 2021, it is inconceivable that the United States would have the highest maternal mortality rate among developed countries with 26.4 deaths per 100,000 live births (Young), given the technological advances in the field of obstetrics and gynecology.

Feminist scholars suggest that when pregnancy became a medicalized event, women lost control of their bodies and the birthing process. Under the guise of providing women with safer conditions, labour and delivery were removed from the purview of midwives and women's only gatherings into hospital settings. Midwives who understood the importance of caring for both the mother and fetus were replaced with physicians more interested in monitoring the fetus. As a result, medical staff placed more emphasis on infant mortality. Consequently, the health needs of mothers took a backseat, and the use of invasive medical procedures, such as C-sections and inducing labour, became common practice. In the last ten years, there has been a growing concern about maternal health and mortality. Every year, in the United States, more than fifty thousand mothers are seriously injured during or after childbirth, and in a four-year study, *USA Today* reporter, Allison Young found that hospitals play a huge role in the culture of negligence that mothers encounter. Young also reports that 60 per cent of hypertension-related strokes and deaths and 90 per cent of deaths associated with hemorrhaging could be prevented if hospital staff had better training and were aware of how much blood a woman loses after giving birth. Although these statistics are shocking, for Black mothers, race adds another layer to the complex problems surrounding maternal health. The National Partnership for Women and Families reports that Black women are three to four times more likely to experience a pregnancy-related death or a preventable maternal death compared with white women (2). It is clear from the statistics that women from all walks of life are dying; however, Black women are dying at a higher rate.

In this chapter, I argue that in addition to hospital negligence when treating early warning signs associated with pregnancy, labour, and birth (such as infection, raised heart rate, or internal bleeding), Black women are dying because of implicit biases rooted in a visual ideology that places them outside the accepted narrative of motherhood. The institution of motherhood and the ideologies surrounding it have an anti-Black sentiment based on the image of the breeder woman and welfare queen. These images affect the risk factors that Black mothers encounter. In my discussion, I draw on the works from scholars of maternal theory and Black feminist theory to critique the power these images have on Black maternal health care.

The Institution of Motherhood in American Culture

Maternal theory scholars analyze motherhood from three perspectives: "motherhood as experience/role, motherhood as institution/ideology, and motherhood as identity/subjectivity" (O'Reilly 203). The institution of American motherhood is a contested space surrounded by the ideologies of patriarchy, technology, and capitalism (Rothman 13). I add that there is a powerful visual ideology that controls the image of who should be a mother and what a mother should look like. Barbara Katz Rothman claims patriarchal control can come in the form of women being pressured to have more children because they are trying for a son, covering for a man's infertility by taking the blame, seeking out insemination alternatives, or having abortion rights controlled (14). In addition to patriarchy, technology as an ideology heavily influences motherhood. The ideology of technology encourages people to think of their bodies as objects that can be controlled like machinery. So in treating the body like a machine, bodily functions and organs are part of a larger system that should operate in a productive and timely manner (Rothman 31). This notion that the human body, if managed properly, can operate like a finely tuned machine extends to pregnancy.

The use of monitoring technologies—such as transvaginal and abdominal ultrasounds, fetal monitors, a host of blood tests, and C-section deliveries—treats mothers like a machine that must deliver a baby in the most efficient, predictable, and rational way possible (Rothman 31). This attitude detaches the woman from the fetus and the physician from the mother. "Birth then becomes something that should happen the same way, each time, for every woman—like how a machine operates—rather than an organic process that has a level of unpre-dictability" (Harper 51). Seeing birth from a technological approach has serious consequences for women because the time needed to give birth becomes controlled by doctors' schedules, hospital costs, and insurance payouts. As a result, doctors can deliver babies without spending arduous amounts of time waiting for the child to arrive. The ideology of technology is tied to capitalism and to this intangible theory that bodies and time are commodities that should be managed.

Capitalism is an ideology that envisions the body as a commodity. As such, mothers and children are looked at for the worth they add to society. The ideologies of patriarchy, technology, and capitalism com-modify a woman's body by valuing her for providing men with sexual intercourse and/or by giving birth. In the context of American capitalism, women of any race could satisfy the sexual urges of men; however, only "healthy white babies" (Rothman 39) were considered precious products to be valued. In her assessment of babies as a commodity, however, Rothman overlooks the commodification of Black mothers and children. When Black women arrived as slaves to the United States, they were situated within the infrastructure of white supremacy's need to protect the economic system of chattel slavery. As such, Black mothers and healthy Black children were considered necessary for the economic growth of the United States.

The final controlling ideology of motherhood is a visual ideology that objectifies the image of a so-called good mom. According to antebellum values of womanhood, a good mom was white, chaste, selfless, caring, and committed to her children and under the protection and care of white patriarchy. Contrarily, this image was used to place Black mothers outside the context of what is considered a good mother. Thus, enslaved Black women were objectified as bad mothers and presented as less than human. Their bodies were meant to be controlled, policed, and used. As a result, they were stereotyped as bad mothers who were sexually promiscuous and incapable of mothering children like white mothers. As such, the written discourse and imagery of Black women as breeders and later welfare queens became part of the country's national narrative (Collins 119). I posit that the breeder woman and welfare queen stereotypes influence the interaction Black mothers have with the medical establishment and the implicit biases they face.

The Breeder Woman and Welfare Mother

The control of Black women's reproductive rights and sexuality was vital to the American economy. Her ability to breed was of great importance to chattel slavery because she was a slave owner's only resource for more slaves (the United States banned the importation of stolen Africans after 1807). Black women were labelled as suitable for having multiple children with any man because she was physically stronger than her white counterpart, and her "animal-like appetite for sex" and reproduction made her an excellent candidate for breeding. As an incentive, pregnant women were assigned lighter loads, given more rations, and sometimes awarded bonuses for giving birth (Collins

51). The breeder woman was responsible for sustaining the slave economy with her womb while also meeting the needs of white men's sexual appetites.

After chattel slavery ended and the United States eventually became an industrial society in the nineteenth and twentieth centuries, Black mothers and children were no longer serving the needs of a plantation economy or providing cheap labour within the unjust system of sharecropping. Black mothers and their children now represented a burden on the economic and social structures of the United States; consequently, the creation of the welfare mother was born. The welfare mother, according to Patricia Hill Collins, is an updated version of the breeder woman, but unlike the breeder woman during slavery who worked, she is satisfied with collecting welfare from the state. Not only is her unemployment an affront to the economic stability of the United States, but it is also the reason politicians cite for controlling her fertility. To make this image believable, politicians created a difference between white and Black unwed mothers. White unwed mothers were categorized as adding worth to American society despite their illegitimate children. The repercussions of her sexual transgressions could be fixed if she were willing to give her child up for adoption. Adoption provided white, middle-class families with a child that could be absorbed into the fabric of white America, hence adding value to society. In contrast, politicians and social workers portrayed Black, unwed mothers, their children, and the Black community negatively.

Unwed Black mothers were characterized as bad mothers who should be punished for creating babies that were "expensive and undesirable" (Solinger 298). And policymakers characterized the Black community as irresponsible and immoral; therefore, they were not assisted or encouraged to place illegitimate children in the adoption system (Solinger 298). It was also commonly believed that Black Americans did not wish to adopt other people's children, which is untrue. Collins suggests that "blood mothers and other mothers" (119) helped care for each other's children, and short-term arrangements often turned into long-term, informal adoptions. White policymakers painted the African American community as a licentious one, which accepted illegitimate children, rather than as a community of people who despite years of abuse and discrimination still maintained the West African value of "community based child care" as a means to survive oppressive living conditions

(Collins 120). Ultimately, the white establishment's attitude criminalized the Black community, and the government pushed the narrative that Black moms were promiscuous, lazy, irresponsible, and unwilling to raise children who would become productive members of society (Collins 76). Without a man (Black or white) to control or provide her with financial support, Black mothers were a threat to white patriarchy and the social and economic fabric of American life. This image is the precursor to the government's justification for controlling Black women's reproductive rights while negating the presence of historical oppression steeped in chattel slavery, Jim Crow, and white supremacy.

The breeder woman and welfare mother have negatively affected how Black motherhood is constructed for the public's consumption and creates a written and visual narrative that demonizes Black mothers and leads to their being dismissed or ignored by medical providers. The dismissal of their concerns causes them to suffer higher rates of complications, subsequently, increasing the maternal mortality rate among Black women. The historically negative images of Black women as breeders and welfare queens play a central role in the racism that Black mothers encounter when dealing with medical professionals and health disparities.

Black Maternal Health and Health Disparities

When it comes to the topic of Black maternal health, most of the research alludes to preexisting health conditions (e.g., weight, diabetes, and heart disease), the mother's age (thirty-five and older), and lifestyle (e.g., alcohol, tobacco, and drugs) as characteristics of high-risk pregnancies. There is also a large body of research that continuously cites access to prenatal care and insurance, socioeconomics, and educational level as disparities affecting Black maternal health, but that simply is not true. After giving birth to her daughter in 2017, tennis star Serena Williams had emergency surgery due to the blood clots she developed in her lungs after explaining to her nurses and doctors about her medical needs. Dr. Shalon Irving and Kira Johnson also suffered complications after giving birth, but neither lived to tell their stories. Irving was a highly educated woman with a PhD in sociology and worked as an epidemiologist at the Centers for Disease Control. Irving died three weeks after giving birth from complications due to hypertension. Johnson was a licensed pilot who spoke five languages and travelled the world. She died twelve hours after delivering her second child via a scheduled C-section at Cedars-Sinai Medical Center in Los Angeles. The fact that Williams had life-threatening difficulties and both Irving and Johnson died dispels the argument that the lack of access to money, insurance, and education are the only risk factors Black mothers face. If the wealthiest and most educated among Black women still face life-threatening complications, then we must explore the effects of racism on Black maternal health.

Dr. Joia Crear-Perry argues that exposure to racism is the real risk factor affecting Black maternal health. I agree with this assessment and note that medical professionals are profoundly affected by implicit biases rooted in the stereotypes of the breeder woman and welfare mother. Because visual literacy is tied to cultural considerations, language and images work together to maintain power relations in society. If we consider the power physicians and nurses have over the choices of Black mothers during labour and then consider the ideological influences that they have been unconsciously conditioned to think about when considering women's bodies and Black women as mothers, then implicit bias becomes a reasonable risk factor for Black women. Black women across the income and educational spectrum face the same life and death outcomes when delivering children, and part of the problem rests with how medical professionals understand the relationship between pain and Black patients.

Black people have been stereotyped as being able to bear physical stress; this is one of the justifications for the extreme labour and abuse they were subjected to during chattel slavery. Black women's experiences within the system of slavery were unique in that they participated in the same strenuous physical labour as men and often while pregnant. They also returned to that same strenuous labour immediately after giving birth, and if they were breeder women, they were required to birth as many children as possible. Out of this discourse grew a belief that Black and white people have biological differences. In a 2016 report on racial bias in pain assessment, Kelly Hoffman et al. found that medical students at various stages in their education and white people in general believe that Black people age at a slower rate, have thicker skin, are more sensitive to smell, are more fertile, and have stronger immune systems than whites do (4296). Additionally, Hoffman et al. report that there is a belief that Black people's blood coagulates more quickly than whites' (4296).

These long-held assumptions are embedded in the medical establishment and affect pain assessment and medication dosages for Black patients, which is one reason why "Black Americans are systematically undertreated for pain relative to white Americans" (Hoffman et al. 4296). This is important to acknowledge because these same assumptions about Black bodies and pain affect how Black mothers are treated when they enter into the world of pregnancy, labour, and delivery—a world heavily influenced and controlled by a white, female, and middle-class narrative of motherhood. Researchers argue that undertreatment is a result of "deeply ingrained unconscious stereotypes about people of color, as well as physicians' difficulty in empathizing with patients whose experiences differ from their own" (Villarosa 20). Valerie Montgomery Rice of Morehouse School of Medicine admits that unconscious biases can influence medical providers when dealing with Black mothers. She has witnessed medical professionals "occasionally withhold epidurals and local anesthetics from African-American women" because they believe Black women have a higher threshold for pain (qtd. in Jones 15). A former labour and delivery nurse, Hakima Payne, was privy to victim-blaming conversations and preconceived ideas about women of colour: "If those people would only do blah, blah, blah, things would be different" (qtd. in Martin and Montagne para. 22). These admissions by medical staff confirm what Black mothers know intuitively—race matters and prejudices exist.

Researchers are finally beginning to explore the relationship between race and implicit bias in the medical establishment. Implicit bias is defined as having an unconscious, negative perception or prejudice against a group of people, such as "minority ethnic populations, immigrants, the poor, low health-literacy individuals, sexual minorities, children, women, the elderly, the mentally ill, the overweight and the disabled" (FitzGerald and Hurst 2). These groups are more likely to encounter implicit biases from medical providers and receive a lower standard of care because of irrelevant traits and immersion in cultures where such groups are portrayed in stereotypical and pejorative ways (FitzGerald and Hurst). Black women face implicit biases due to the images of the breeder woman and welfare mother. These negative stereotypes combined with the belief that Black bodies can endure more pain have created a culture of neglect for Black mothers. As a result, this culture contributes to high maternal complications and deaths in Black mothers. William Hall et al. suggest that bias takes many forms during patient-doctor interactions. The most damaging expression is that of a "dominant and condescending tone that decreases the likelihood that patients will feel heard and valued by their providers and receive more or less through diagnostic work for patients of color" (Hall et al. 2). With the current emphasis on Black maternal health in the news, more Black mothers are coming forward with their stories of dismissal and bias. For example, Tai Haden-Moore repeatedly told medical staff that something was amiss and that her stomach felt heavier than normal. Her concerns were not taken seriously until she ended up in the bathroom with blood gushing everywhere. In this case, her physician did not trust her instincts and chose not to intervene early. Consequently, she had an emergency C-section. Haden-Moore suggests that her treatment was because she was Black, and even though nothing directly racist was said to her, she feels that medical staff do not show the same concern for Black mothers. She states: "I feel like they always diminish us and think that we're complaining too much, or asking too many questions, or we're drug-seeking ... those types of things" (qtd. in Pearson 3). Annett Brooks echoes Haden-Moore's opinion: "I would like for [care providers] to be culturally sensitive to the black female experience and to recognize and check their own biases. I want them to treat us with the same care and concern that they show white women and children" (qtd. in Pearson 6).

Creating a more diverse healthcare workforce can help alleviate some of the implicit biases Black mothers face, but that is a long-term fix to a problem that has immediate consequences. My suggestion is that medical staff participate in courses that discuss implicit bias and visual imagery. If medical staff can see how stereotypes like the breeder woman and welfare queen can unconsciously affect their opinion of Black mothers, they may be able to reconsider the decisions they make when providing care. The high maternal mortality rate and the anecdotal experiences of Black women are an indication that health professionals need to train medical professionals to recognize their own implicit biases so that all mothers can live to raise their children.

Works Cited

Collins, Patricia Hill. *Black Feminist Thought: Knowledge Consciousness, and the Politics of Empowerment*. Routledge, 1991.

Crear-Perry, Joia. "Race Isn't a Risk Factor in Maternal Health. Racism Is." *Rewire News*, Apr. 11 2018, rewire.news/article/2018/04/11/maternal-health-replace-race-with-racism/. Accessed 22 Mar. 2021.

FitzGerald, Chloë, and Samia Hurst. "Implicit Bias in Healthcare Professionals: A Systematic Review." *BMC Medical Ethics*, vol. 18, no. 1, 2017, p. 19, doi:10.1186/s12910-017-0179-8.

Hall, William J. et al. "Implicit Racial/Ethnic Bias Among Health Care Professionals and Its Influence on Health Care Outcomes: A Sys-tematic Review" *American Journal of Public Health* vol. 105, no. 12, 2015, pp. 60-76.

Hoffman, Kelly, et al. "Racial Bias in Pain Assessment and Treatment Recommendations, and False Beliefs about Biological Differences Between Blacks and Whites." *Proceedings of the National Academy of Sciences of the United States of America*, vol. 113, no. 16, 2016, pp. 4296-4301.

Harper, Kimberly. *The Ethos of Black Motherhood in America. Only White Women Get Pregnant*. Lexington Books, 2020.

Jones, Rachel. "Why Giving Birth in the US is Surpisingly Deadly." *National Geographic*, Jan. 2019, www.nationalgeographic.com/magazine/article/giving-birth-in-united-states-suprisingly-deadly. Accessed 22 Mar. 2021.

Martin, Nina, and Renee Montagne. "Black Mothers Keep Dying After Giving Birth, Shalon Irving's Story Explains Why." *NPR*, Dec. 7 2017, www.npr.org/2017/12/07/568948782/black-mothers-keep-dying-after-giving-birth-shalon-irvings-story-explains-why. Accessed 22 Mar. 2021.

O'Reilly, Andrea. *Maternal Theory: Essential Readings*. Demeter Press, 2007.

Rothman, Barbara Katz. *Recreating Motherhood*. Rutgers University Press, 2000.

Pearson, C. "Black Women Face More Trauma during Childbirth." *The Huffington Post*, 18 June 2018, www.huffingtonpost.com/entry/

black-women-childbirth-mortality-trauma_us_5b045eaae4b0784 cd2af0f71. Accessed 5 Apr. 2021.

Solinger, Rickie. "Race and 'Value': Black and White Illegitimate Babies, 1945-1965." *Mothering Ideology, Experience, and Agency*, edited by Evelyn Nakano Glenn, Grace Chang, and Linda Rennie Forcey, Routledge, 1994, pp. 287-310.

Villarosa, Linda. "Why America's Black Mothers and Babies Are in a Life-or-Death Crisis." *New York Times*, Apr. 11 2018, www.nytimes. com/2018/04/11/magazine/black-mothers-babies-death-maternal-mortality. html?mtrref=undefined&gwh=799DAE8E4080CE5 4CB9 0F1A9240D 868B&gwt=pay. Accessed 22 Mar. 2021.

Young, Allison. "Hospitals Know How to Protect Mothers. They Just Aren't Doing It." *USA Today*, July 26 2018, www.usatoday.com/in-depth/news/investigations/deadly-deliveries/2018/07/26/maternal-mortality-rates-preeclampsia-postpartum-hemorrhage-safety/ 546889002/. Accessed 22 Mar. 2021.

Chapter 2

Family and Family Practice: The Mothering in Family Medicine

Arundhati Dhara

The face of family medicine is changing. Or, rather, it has already changed. Gone is the image of the greying male doctor, on call to a community at all hours of the day, doling out medical advice to grateful patients. After a rewarding day saving lives, he came home to a hot meal cooked by his loving wife and the smiles of his adoring children. He has been replaced by me, a mother of three who spends her days zipping between clinical gigs. I come home to take calls from the hospital or clinic while cooking dinner. My partner, equally frazzled and exhausted by his own career, supervises baths and homework and tries (with limited success) to referee the catastrophic demise of a Lego tower.

My experiences as a mother and a family physician and the data surrounding gender and primary care have convinced me that the feminization of medicine and the expectations of how we deliver care are related. In this chapter, I reflect on the ways that traditional models of paternalistic and directive care have been replaced with practices of medicine that reflect modern motherhood. Family physicians, increasingly women, are tasked with transferring their socialized feminine roles from the home to the office. I will also consider the phenomenon of burnout through my experience as a practicing physician and frame it in gendered terms in family medicine.

This chapter is not meant to suggest that family medicine does not also hold in its ranks extraordinary men or that our practice is or ought to be confined to certain settings. I should also be clear that as a professional physician, my approach to medicine reflects my years of training. By contrast, my experience with motherhood is more ill-defined, since it is almost entirely made up along the way (as I imagine it is for every parent). I am therefore not an expert, and my ideas come from one who is living the experience rather than as a scholar. What I offer here are my own observations of the considerable overlap—not all of it positive—between the skills and pressures of family life on the one hand and the practice of family medicine on the other.

The Practice of Family Medicine Is Changing: Reflections on My Personal Practice

I completed family medicine residency in 2011. I used my position to travel rural and remote regions of Canada, experiment with different practices and lifestyles, and learn new clinical skills. Much of my practice was hospital based and very specific: emergency and inpatient medicine, addictions, and palliative care. At the same time, I was aware that this was not what I was supposed to do. My training emphasized the opposite of the nomadic existence I had created; family doctors are meant to be stable and create long-term relationships with their patients and the communities they serve. When asked by other doctors when I would "settle down and join a practice" I would explain that I was only trying to determine where I would set up a clinic, when the reality was that I was enjoying not having to maintain protracted relationships with patients.

It was only after I became pregnant myself that I began to explore a permanent practice, adding the responsibilities of parenthood to those of a so-called real family doctor. It did not feel organic. My decisions have been difficult. In fact, my transition to a traditional family practice most closely resembles the journey to step-motherhood described by the anthropologist Pam Downe—it has been a deliberate and slow process. She describes a "first trimester" of step-motherhood, full of ambivalence and uncertainty. I experienced similar feelings towards traditional practice, doing short-term locums and rejecting the relationships that define family medicine

With pregnancy and family life, I could no longer work shifts in the emergency room, looking after inpatients overnight, or otherwise be away from a new baby. Nor did my new domestic arrangement allow for me to be gone for weeks at a time to travel to remote communities. Moreover, and much to my chagrin, I found I did not want to miss bedtimes and early morning snuggles with my children. As I adopted the role of biological mother, I entered what Downe describes as the second and third "trimesters" in her journey towards becoming a step-mother. I fell for family medicine, as Downe did for her family, and I began to see the value that its relationships bring to patients. Finally, I internalized the gendered care and nurture Downe describes as the "third trimester" in becoming an "other-mother" (Downe 31).

Thus, my experience of adopting a family practice was anchored in and precipitated by adopting the responsibilities of motherhood. As I went about the work of redefining my personal identities, I became more and more aware of the divergence between traditional notions of family doctors and the realities I saw in myself and those around me.

FIFE-ing and Whole Person Care: How Family Medicine Mediates Lego Tower Catastrophes

Rather than focusing solely on a disease state, modern family medicine adopts a whole-person approach, in which empathy is crucial for not only eliciting information but also healing the patient. The centrality of the physician-patient relationship is codified as one of the four guiding principles of family medicine ("Principles").

By the time I was in residency, whole-person approaches were part of the formal curriculum, with the physician acting in an advisory role rather than providing prescriptive actions regarding health. As I have developed my practice in medicine, I have been struck at how much of good doctoring has paralleled good mothering. In fact, it has never been clear to me which was the chicken and which the egg: Am I a good mother because I am a good doctor or is it the other way around?

There's a running joke among physicians when faced with a patient who does not seem to have a clear medical complaint or for one whose symptoms simply do not add up: "Did you FIFE them?" FIFE is an acronym for feelings, ideas, fears, and expectations. The goal is to figure out the root of the patient's problem—physical, psychological, or some combination thereof. It is incredibly awkward to elicit this information from patients early in training, and we mock the concept to hide our clumsiness. But by the time family physicians are fully trained, FIFE-ing is an invaluable diagnostic tool for some of our most challenging cases.

During my own training, a woman came in to get a form filled out for insurance to cover her orthotics. It was a simple appointment, but something felt wrong, and eventually the woman disclosed years of spousal abuse. The ability to move beyond the ostensible reason for a visit to the root of a problem is the real utility of the sometimes ridiculed FIFE principle.

Strangely, I think of that woman often when dealing with my toddler. Increased frequency of bathroom accidents and meltdowns over the inevitable collapse of Lego towers almost always results in a conversation validating the frustrations of a three-year-old and participating in long, rambling (often incoherent) FIFE sessions that might result in a snuggle, a story, and hopefully a small step on the path to my child's development.

Relational Care in Motherhood and Medicine

Family medicine has embraced relational skills as central to its practice alongside academic rigour. A 2008 report by the College of Family Physicians called "Rethinking Undergraduate Medical Education" takes pains to differentiate family medicine from other specialties, exhorting medical educators to focus on interprofessional team-based care and being present for patients in the care process (Weston et al. 23).

In fact, women family doctors are more likely to enter team-based care arrangements over men (Coyle et al. 267), and their practice styles closely align with the College's recommendations. The way women practice family medicine is a mix of using empathy, asking the right questions, and offering their time (Roter and Hall 510).

The same can be said of modern mothering. There is an endless stream of traditional and social media telling us that we must listen more to our children, that we should see the world through their eyes, and that to do this we need to spend more time with them. And indeed, we do spend more time in childcare today than our mothers did ("Parents Spend Time"), despite the fact that women also clock more hours working outside the home and fathers have increased their own share of childcare (Houle et al.).

Women family physicians are thus tasked with Herculean feats of being there for others: more time with patients, more time with children and full presence in both spheres. The reality is I simply cannot do it, and I confess to feeling a great deal of guilt. Society expects me to want to spend ever more quality time with my children and as a good doctor to listen intently to my patients for as long as they need me. The resulting emotional exhaustion is a tinderbox, ready for a bad day to spark a raging burnout fire.

The Patient Medical Home and the Third Shift

There is a calendar in my house without which my family would fall apart. Dinner menus, birthdays, and dentist appointments are all carefully coordinated. I am constantly planning and organizing, thinking about making next week's meals or volunteering at school. At the office, I function as my patient's "medical home" ("Patient Medical Home"), acting as a clearinghouse for health-related presentations, offering access to allied health and specialists and coordinating care between various silos. It means I can never stop organizing my family life or the care of my patients, and the weight of the combined load is immense.

At least in the home, this mental work is sometimes called the "third shift." Performed after the paid workday (the first shift) and the responsibilities of child and family care (the second shift), this work falls disproportionately to mothers. It includes the strategizing and anticipation of tasks to make family life function (Robertson et al. 191), and it has been largely invisible until recently, when public conversations about its importance have begun.

But in the office, this work remains hidden. Perhaps because patients are often not present when phone calls are made and letters are reviewed, they may not understand it as work. Certainly, it is not remunerated by provincial insurers in traditional fee-for-service compensation models— it is taken as a matter of course in the practice of family medicine. Payment is for the clinical encounter alone. In both the home and the office, this work simply ensures that daily life and practice continue. It is labour without a tangible product, and as such it just does not count.

Burnout and Self Care: You Are Not Good Enough

The concept of physician burnout has had increasing traction in recent years; it is characterized by emotional exhaustion and affects those with perfectionistic tendencies who ultimately feel as though they have not accomplished their goals (Patel et al. 98). Ultimately, burnout leads to disengagement from work and life. Discussions of physician burnout have focussed on the long hours of critical-care physicians as well as feelings of helplessness as patients lie sick or dying. And although all this is certainly true, there is a far more pedestrian truth we have not yet grappled with as a profession: Being a female family doctor is a risk factor for experiencing burnout (Lemire 480).

There is a pervasive and insidious narrative that tells mothers and family doctors they are not good enough: They need to work harder and do more. I attended a town hall recently in which the health minister attributed the shortage of family doctors to younger physicians looking for "work-life balance." Given the context and environment, those of us in the audience presumed he meant that women were taking time away from medicine for their families. The concept of balance is an interesting one for physician mothers, with both roles demanding a complete sublimation of personal identities into the role. For physicians, this takes the form of professionalism and caring for patients. Regardless of what else might be going on, it becomes impossible to escape our responsibilities to patients. In fact, physicians most likely to experience burnout are those whose work drive leads them to have no balance between work and other parts of their lives (Patel et al. 98). For mothers, the story is similar. Our personal desires are no longer relevant, or they must merge with our children's (Thurer 335).Women general practitioners specifically cite emotional exhaustion as the cause of their burnout (Houkes et al. 10), and surely the inability to reconcile these two care roles is a factor.

Perhaps to enforce our adherence to these norms, we are also offered social and political narratives of our inadequacy and laziness. Family doctors are told over and over that the solution to the physician shortage is that we ought to work more (Boissinot), and the media is rife with stories of bad medical outcomes, frequently implicating the lack of a family physician or that the doctor did not listen to the patient.

In studies of parental burnout, mothers cite the fear of not being good enough as a significant factor (Hubert and Aujoulat 4). We have set mothers up with outsize power (Thurer, 335); the entire outcome of their children's lives is pinned on the love and care of mothers. The combined effects of motherhood and medicine can be crushing.

There are now programs in residencies across Canada dedicated to physician wellness, and it has even been taken up as a primary cause by the Canadian Medical Association. But perhaps to maintain a veneer of gender neutrality, there is no substantive discussion about how gender and medicine, especially in woman-dominated family medicine, are connected to burnout. Indeed, the 2019 residency match follows a recent trend of high numbers of vacant family medicine spots (Collier), suggesting that medical students are not choosing the discipline. In the face of Canada's shortage of family doctors, it is critical that we confront the gendered reality of the practise of family medicine.

A Way Forward

It has become clear to me over the years that I made the right choice to specialize in family medicine. I have the freedom to pursue a variety of professional and personal goals. But in becoming a mother, I have also realized that the work of family medicine recalls the work of the home. The way that I run my practice parallels the way I mother—in how I approach problems and the types of labour I perform for my family and my patients. But perhaps not so surprising are the ways that this work is invisible and unrewarded in both contexts, as there is a long history of undervaluing women's work. Professionally, this means that women family doctors experience burnout and that medical students, perhaps sensing these feelings, are not choosing family medicine. Personally, it means that I just do not have it in me to help my son rebuild his Lego tower, and that makes me angry and sad.

Even though the medical community and politicians have had many panicked conversations about Canada's lack of family doctors, relatively little attention has been paid to the gender dynamics at play. It is time to start that uncomfortable dialogue for the good of our families and for the good of family practice.

Works Cited

Boissinot, Jacques. "Quebec Doctors Aren't Taking on Enough Patients, Gaétan Barrette Says." *Montreal Gazette*, 4 Oct. 2016, montrealgazette.com/news/quebec/family-doctors-arent-signing-up-enough-patients-health-minister. Accessed 22 Mar. 2021.

Coyle, Natalie, et al. "Characteristics of Physicians and Patients Who Join Team-Based Primary Care Practices: Evidence from Quebec's Family Medicine Groups." *Health Policy*, vol. 116, no. 2-3, 2014, pp. 264-72.

Collier, Roger. "Family Medicine Again Dominates Unfilled Positions in Residency Match." *CMAJ News*, cmajnews.com/2019/02/28/ family-medicine-again-dominates-unfilled-positions-in-residency-match-cmaj-109-5727/. Accessed 22 Mar. 2021.

Downe, Pamela J. Stepping on Maternal Ground: Reflections on Becoming an "Other-Mother". *Journal of the Motherhood Initiative for Research and Community Involvement,* vol. 15, no. 1, 2001, pp. 28-40.

Houkes, Inge, et al. "Development of Burnout over Time and the Causal Order of the Three Dimensions of Burnout among Male and Female GPs. A Three-Wave Panel Study." *BMC Public Health*, BioMed Central, 18 Apr. 2011, www.ncbi.nlm.nih.gov/pubmed /21501467. Accessed 22 Mar. 2021.

Houle, Patricia, et al. "Spotlight on Canadians: Results from the General Social Survey Changes in Parents' Participation in Domestic Tasks and Care for Children from 1986 to 2015." *Changes in Parents' Participation in Domestic Tasks and Care for Children from 1986 to 2015*, 7 June 2017, www150.statcan.gc.ca/n1/pub/89-652-x/89-652-x2017001-eng.htm. Accessed 22 Mar. 2021.

Hubert, Sarah, and Isabelle Aujoulat. "Parental Burnout: When Exhausted Mothers Open Up." *Frontiers in Psychology*, Frontiers Media S.A., 26 June 2018, www.ncbi.nlm.nih.gov/pmc/articles/ PMC6028779/.

Lemire, Francine. "Combating Physician Burnout." *The College of Family Physicians of Canada*, The College of Family Physicians of Canada, 1 June 2018, www.cfp.ca/content/64/6/480#ref-1.

"Parents Now Spend Twice as Much Time with Their Children as 50 Years Ago." *The Economist*, The Economist Newspaper, 27 Nov. 2017, www.economist.com/graphic-detail/2017/11/27/parents-now-spend-twice-as-much-time-with-their-children-as-50-years-ago.

Patel, Rikinkumar S. et al. "Factors Related to Physician Burnout and Its Consequences: A Review." *Behavioral Sciences* (Basel, Switzerland), MDPI, 25 Oct. 2018, www.ncbi.nlm.nih.gov/pmc/articles/PMC6262585/. Accessed 22 Mar. 2021.

"Principles." *The College of Family Physicians of Canada*, www.cfpc.ca/principles/. Accessed 22 Mar. 2021.

Robertson, Lindsey G., et al. "Mothers and Mental Labor: A Phenomenological Focus Group Study of Family-Related Thinking Work - Lindsey G. Robertson, Tamara L. Anderson, M. Elizabeth Lewis Hall, Christina Lee Kim, 2019." *SAGE Journals*, journals.sagepub.com/doi/abs/10.1177/0361684319825581. Accessed 22 Mar. 2021.

Roter, Debra L., and Judith A. Hall. "Physician Gender and Patient-Centered Communication: A Critical Review of Empirical Research." *Annual Review of Public Health*, vol. 25, no. 1, 2004, pp. 497-519., doi:10.1146/annurev.publhealth.25.101802.123134.

"The Patient's Medical Home." *The College of Family Physicians of Canada*, www.cfpc.ca/pmh/. Accessed 22 Mar. 2021.

Weston, Wayne, et al. Rethinking Undergraduate Medical Education: A View from Family Medicine. *CFPC*, 28 Apr. 2008 www.cfpc.ca/uploadedFiles/Education/VIEW%20FROM%20FAMILY%20MEDICINE_Final%20April2008(1).pdf. Accessed 22 Mar. 2021.

Chapter 3

"And Who Are You?" One Chinese Mother's Journey from Advocating for Her Children to Maternal Empowerment

Catherine Ma

As a mother, my experiences with physicians have transformed me from being a silent consumer to staunch advocate for my children. This form of maternal empowerment in which mothers take on the role of healthcare advocate, partner up with physicians to find the best treatment options, and actively manage the progression of their children's illness is an important topic to discuss because it offers women the opportunity to validate the frustrations and disappointments of dealing with the medical community. Prior to becoming a mother, I fit those Chinese stereotypes of being quiet, meek, and demure, but motherhood has acted as a catalyst to help me find my voice. Using my voice often surprises many physicians, as it defies their Chinese stereotypes when I am outspoken and perform motherhood with a sense of urgency when I feel my children's safety or health is at risk. In many ways, I become an expert on their conditions to properly advocate for the best treatment options, which is not new as many parents are pressured to become both advocate and medical expert when their child's health comes into question (Mulligan et al. 322). It is never easy to challenge a doctor's misdiagnosis or stand up to a physician who pressures you to agree to surgery when you are unsure, but these unpleasant experiences taught me two valuable lessons—that my voice is powerful and my research skills are quite useful. I was never one to question physicians when it came to my own health, but since becoming a mother, I have learned how to become a strong advocate for not just my children but my entire family. Now I use the power of my voice to ask those difficult questions that challenge the authority of physicians that most people shirk because doctors continue to be heralded as gods. I am often asked by my children's doctors, "And who are you?" when I ask my list of questions. Carl Dunst and his colleagues found medical professionals often blamed family members or construed them to be problematic when they asked questions regarding the physician's treatment protocol ("Enabling and Empowering Families" 76). As a mother, I need the physician's expertise to be factual and clear, so many of my questions reflect that nature, but I also am interested in the way they respond to my questions. Are they condescending? Do they respect my child and speak to them with a genuine and caring nature? Are they rattled by my questions? These are all aspects that fall under my maternal radar that will affect my decision to choose this individual as my child's care provider. I simply want a physician who is caring and knowledgeable, respects me and my child, is unafraid to say that they do not know but will find out, is trustworthy, and works just as hard as I do to provide the best care for my children. My chapter chronicles the importance of using one's voice to navigate through the United States healthcare system and hopefully inspire other mothers to find their voice.

My first transformative experience with a physician began with my daughter who was born with a preauricular cyst. This genetic condition results in malformed sinus tracts located just underneath the skin near the outer ear ("What Are Preauricular Pits?"). In my daughter's case, the tiny pinhole cyst became repeatedly infected leading to an abscess, which we would drain with warm compresses. She needed surgery to remove this cyst that was close to her facial nerve, and if done incorrectly, she could lose her ability to smile and move her facial muscles on that side of her face. Being first-time parents, my partner and I found this experience particularly stressful because we were not completely sure how to deal with this situation and worried about the potential damage to her face. Our paediatrician was able to get us a same-day appointment with a local otolaryngologist, who diagnosed her as having a branchial cleft cyst that would require surgery to correct. After hearing his diagnosis, I scoured through the internet to read up on branchial cleft cysts, and the location of them, usually by the neck, did not seem to match where my daughter's infection was situated, which was closer to the front of her outer ear (Boringi 125). Being a trained researcher, I pored through numerous medical journals until I found out that she had a preauricular cyst. I wanted to question this doctor regarding his diagnosis, but my husband told me that was not a good idea because he was a physician and knew better than us. Little did I know at the time how this physician adhered to the traditional expert model, in which he assumed that his expertise was the only knowledge that was considered valuable (Brookman-Frazee 197). If I had kept silent, this doctor would have operated on the wrong part of my child. When I look back on this experience, I can still feel the anger rising within me with what had transpired at our follow-up appointment. I had made copies of all my medical journal articles to show this doctor what I had found and was respectful when I politely asked if my daughter might have a pre-auricular cyst instead of a branchial cleft cyst. I expected him to review my findings with an open mind, but what I really wanted to tell him was that he had clearly misdiagnosed her. What transpired was something I had not anticipated. He verbally attacked me; he called me overprotective, said I was overreacting, dismissed my research, and probably could not understand why I would challenge his diagnosis. Proponents of these expert models tend to regard the information families hold as inconsequential and often make decisions regarding diagnoses and treatment with little, if any, input from the family (Dunst et al., "Family-Oriented Program" 221). I was surprised at his outburst, but his behavior taught me that there is power in my voice, and my knowledge in research helped prevent a medical mishap from occurring. That was the day that changed the way I viewed all medical professionals, and I began to choose physicians who took a more collaborative approach to medicine in treating my loved ones. Unfortunately, not all professionals recognize the value of collaborating with families and how this collaboration improves patient outcomes (DeChillo, Koren, and Schultz 574).

Our paediatrician at the time was one who valued my judgment as a mother, researcher, psychologist, and professor. He truly listened to my concerns regarding my children's health and understood that any

decisions regarding their health were up to me. His role as our paediatrician was to provide his expertise in paediatrics because I did not
share his knowledge. He would often joke that he has to say what he has
to say because he is a paediatrician, but he also knew that I may not
always follow his suggestions. In addition, he respected my decisions to
pick and choose which advice to follow as it fit my children's needs.
Proponents of these family-focused models of healthcare that centre on
mutual respect are more in line with the type of professional I want to
treat my children. That otolaryngologist only cared about his own
opinions and diagnoses without considering the valuable expertise
mothers have regarding their children. Professionals who employ a
collective approach with their patient's parents tend to experience more
positive health outcomes for their patients, but this change can only be
achieved if the physician recognizes the expertise of the parents regarding
their children and is secure enough to understand that by sharing
knowledge to empower parents, their expertise as a medical provider
does not lessen (DeChillo, Koren, and Schultz 574-75). Based on that
otolaryngologist's verbal outburst, I knew we would not be returning to
him for any further treatment due to his unprofessionalism. During that
time, I was fortunate to be a member of an online mothers support group
and had posted a message asking its members if any of their children
had preauricular cysts. By the end of the day, I had found another mother
who lived nearby whose child had the same condition, and we quickly
became acquainted online to share our experiences. It was her paediatric
otolaryngologist who eventually performed my daughter's surgery to
correct her condition. I quickly learned how powerful mothers were in
creating their own supportive networks. With the advent of the internet,
mothers can reach out for support, and this can be empowering for many
women. As a researcher who specializes in breastfeeding, I pay it forward
by offering support and my expertise to a local online group of nursing
mothers. Providing that service helps numerous women overcome the
challenges of breastfeeding and motherhood that often go unnoticed by
many medical professionals. It is the sharing of these maternal experiences that can lessen the marginalization many mothers often feel when
they are dismissed by the medical community.

The second experience that shaped my view of physicians occurred
when my older son was diagnosed with severe sleep apnea at the age of
five. My husband had noticed that his breathing would often stop as he

slept, and he would jolt up to catch his breath. We took the initiative and asked our paediatrician to have our son sleep tested. During the consultation with a new otolaryngologist, we learned that a sleep number of five to fourteen is considered a mild respiratory disturbance, fifteen to thirty is considered moderate, and a number above thirty is considered severe apnea. My son's number was eighty-three. This was quite alarming but as I diligently took down notes from the office visit, I noticed that he was a young doctor and fresh out of medical school. So when he seemed eager to schedule surgery to remove his enlarged tonsils and adenoids, this set off a red flag for me, as I wanted to discuss our options, seek a second opinion, and sleep on it before making such a big decision. What alarmed me the most was how he casually mentioned that with severe cases of apnea, pulmonary edema can result postoperatively because the resistance from the tonsils is gone, which often results in the collapse of the lungs. This was due to the change in flow and pressure difference, in which removing the resistance (e.g., enlarged tonsils) can cause a flow of fluids into the lungs. If this happens, the only solution is to intubate and medicate him with diuretics to get rid of the fluid. I asked him how often that happens, and he told me that he witnessed the edema in three adults and once in a twelve-year-old child. He must have felt my hesitation in having him perform the surgery with this potential complication, as he mentioned that if we go somewhere else for the surgery, we need to make sure they have a paediatric intensive care unit (PICU) for the first night and adequate support staff. The only words I heard were intubation and PICU, which worried me. As with many mothers, I read up on the research on sleep apnea and quickly learned that this condition was linked with heightened hypertension, heart disease, attention problems, behavioural problems in school, not getting enough rest/REM sleep, and growth problems in children (Gozal 103-06; Tan et al. 115-16). I also knew that my son did not fit that profile. He was happy, did not exhibit any behavioural problems, was doing well in school, had no problems growing, was attentive in class, was loved by his teachers, and had normal blood pressure based on his last physical. I also knew that there was a chance that he would outgrow his apnea as his body caught up with the size of his tonsils.

What concerned me was knowing how the postoperative complications could present a more serious and immediate health threat. My two gravest concerns were how would he react to the general anaesthesia and whether he would he get edema in his lungs and need to be intubated. I was also worried about him suffering from additional, potentially life-threatening, complications from surgery or contracting something worse from being in a hospital. I knew I was afraid of the tonsillectomy and adenoidectomy that this doctor was pressuring me to schedule. The last thing he mentioned was that we would need to get an evaluation from a paediatric pulmonologist which prompted me to find the best one in New York City, and this is how we found an alternative to surgery. The physician I found was a board-certified paediatric pulmonologist at New York-Presbyterian Morgan Stanley Children's Hospital, and when we scheduled our consultation, I noticed that she accepted both private and public insurance. This may not seem like much of a difference to others, but to me, it was evidence that this doctor was dedicated to caring for all her patients. Prior to meeting with her, we had met with another paediatric otolaryngologist who was a top expert in his field. He pioneered a procedure where he shaved the tonsils as opposed to completely removing them. His procedure was less painful, entailed less blood loss, and had a quicker recovery time. The only downside was that he did not accept our insurance, and as a matter of fact, he did not accept any insurance. This revelation highlighted to me how flawed the American medical system is, as access to excellent medical care is largely determined in part by one's financial situation. Imagine being a parent whose child needed a life-saving surgery, but they had to pick and choose who would operate on their child not based on the skill of the surgeon but their ability to pay for their child's medical bills.

Our family is not rich, but if we chosen this doctor, we would have saved up and found a way to pay for his services, but it left a bad taste in my mouth, as his billing policy clearly segregated those who could afford his services and those who could not. I may be idealistic and naïve in my beliefs in paediatric surgeons, but how can a doctor who specializes in helping children only care to help those whose parents could afford him? Dealing with this doctor seemed so problematic on multiple levels, but I was fortunate to have found a different doctor who reignited my hope. We told her of our plan to try continuous positive airway pressure (CPAP) on our five-year-old. She was not convinced, as she had never come across a situation in which parents requested CPAP, and she was unsure about whether a young child could be compliant enough to be on CPAP with the restrictiveness of wearing a mask to sleep while air is forced into their airways. Luciana Palombini, Rafael Pelayo, and Christian Guilleminault, however, have found that CPAP treatment can be an effective nonsurgical option for sleep-related breathing disorders (e414).

Even though the paediatrician was unfamiliar with the logistics of our plan, she was open-minded enough to listen to us and help us in any way that she could. In all my dealings with physicians, I have noticed that the best ones truly listen to their patients and their parents. They do not hold a god complex, in which they view that they are the only voices that matter in deciding what is best for their patients. They work together with the parents to find the best solution for their patient, and this begins by truly listening to the parents. This doctor took the time to help us navigate through the confusing maze of CPAP distributors and our insurance company. When the CPAP supplier she recommended did not accept our insurance plan, she and her staff worked tirelessly to find one that did. She helped us troubleshoot and answered all my emails to problem solve situations as they arose. I am always so grateful for doctors who answer emails because they could easily bill us for their time or ask us to make an appointment to discuss the issues in person. In the span of eleven months, our son was compliant with his CPAP, and he eventually grew into his tonsils as we had predicted. This experience showed us the importance of advocating for our children and finding doctors who were willing to try new treatment options that they were unfamiliar with.

My experiences with both my children provide critical exemplars of the role of maternal voices in medical advocacy. In many ways, mothers play a crucial role in how they know their children on a more personal level than any physician, which makes them an expert to their children. In addition, the medical research that mothers have access to on the internet gives them formidable power in how they can discuss treatment options with their child's medical providers. Sadly, a major obstacle in leveling the medical playing field is how physicians view the role of mothers, as many take an expert-oriented approach as opposed to a collaborative one. Many physicians still feel threatened by the expertise that mothers hold. Yet they should understand the power of mothers not as a threat to their status but as a valuable resource in facilitating the best patient outcomes (DeChillo, Koren, and Schultz 575). With the growing responsibility of mothers to become medical experts and advocates for their children, how do we learn to channel the power of our voices? I believe that the first step towards this new model of mothering stems from sharing maternal experiences on a variety of levels in medicine. This step can change the way future physicians are trained and dramatically redistribute the power in the medical community to be shared between parents and physicians.

These parent-professional partnerships focus on the joint benefits of parents and physicians working together and using their expertise to find the best treatment options for the patient (Brookman-Frazee 197). An increasing amount of research finds that professionals who employ a collective approach with parents of children dealing with health concerns often results in more positive outcomes for their young patients, but this change can only be achieved if the professional recognizes and values the expertise parents have regarding their children (DeChillo, Koren, and Schultz 574). Lastly, it is also important to acknowledge my privilege, as I have the flexibility in my work schedule to find the best doctors, the finances to consult with top experts, the added benefits of private healthcare insurance, the time to do the necessary research, the education to understand medical jargon, and the access to expensive peer-reviewed medical journals. Low-income families may not have these tools to support the best health outcomes for their children, as evidenced by some physicians who do not accept any insurance to offset medical costs. This is the reason why literature that exposes these marginalized experiences must be brought out into the open so we can further challenge this medical paradigm and move closer towards parent-physician relationships that are based more on equity and inclusion.

Works Cited

Boringi, Mamatha, et al. "Branchial Cleft Cyst—A Case Report with Review of Literature." *Journal of Orofacial Sciences*, vol. 6, no. 2, 2014, pp. 125-28.

Brookman-Frazee, Lauren. "Using Parent/Clinician Partnerships in Parent Education Programs for Children with Autism." *Journal of Positive Behavior Interventions*, vol. 6, no. 4, 2004, pp. 195-213.

"What Are Preauricular Pits?" *Children's Hospital of Philadelphia*, 7 Mar. 2019, www.chop.edu/conditions-diseases/preauricular-pits. Accessed 23 Mar. 2021.

DeChillo, Neal, Paul E. Koren, and Kathryn H. Schultze. "From Paternalism to Partnership: Family and Professional Collaboration in Children's Mental Health." *American Journal of Orthopsychiatry*, vol. 64, no. 4, 1994, pp. 564-76.

Dunst, Carl J., et al. "Family-Oriented Program Models and Professional Helpgiving Practices." *Family Relations*, vol. 51, no. 3, 2002, pp. 221-29.

Dunst, Carl J., et al. "Enabling and Empowering Families of Children with Health Impairments." *Children's Health Care,* vol. 17, no. 2, 1988, pp. 71-81.

Gozal, David. "Obstructive Sleep Apnea in Children: Implications for the Developing Central Nervous System." *Seminars in Pediatric Neurology*, vol. 15, no. 2, 2008, pp. 100-06.

Mulligan, Janice, et al. "Transparency, Hope, and Empowerment: A Model for Partnering with Parents of a Child with Autism Spectrum Disorder at Diagnosis and Beyond." *Social Work in Mental Health,* vol. 10, no. 4, 2012, pp. 311-30.

Palombini, Luciana, Rafael Pelayo, and Christian Guilleminault. "Efficacy of Automated Continuous Positive Airway Pressure in Children with Sleep-Related Breathing Disorders in an Attended Setting." *Pediatrics*, vol. 113, no. 5, 2004, pp. e412-17.

Tan, Hui-Leng et al. "Obstructive Sleep Apnea in Children: A Critical Update." *Nature and Science of Sleep,* vol. 5, 2013, pp. 109-23.

Chapter 4

Untrustworthy Bodies

Ariel Watson

My labour began with a violation, a small tearing not just of flesh but of boundaries and trust. My doctor seemed surprised at each of the last few meetings I had with her when I expressed a fervent disinclination to being induced. In Nova Scotia, we had been buried by weekly blizzards the entirety of my third trimester; in January, our car and plow got stuck at the bottom of our steep eight-hundred-foot driveway in a snowstorm, and from then until April, I trekked ten minutes up or down the icy slope every day to get to work, snow up to my shoulders on either side, dragging my work and groceries on a toboggan behind me. I was desperately afraid that the baby would come early, that I would find myself climbing down the hill between contractions or watched by two wary cats as I delivered alone in my house in the middle of the woods. I worked right up until the end, the baby due to arrive at the same time as the semester ended at the university where I taught. At 3:00 a.m. on the morning of my due date, I was finishing edits on an overdue article. I had nightmares that I would be in the hospital, still marking student papers as nurses knotted me into a paper gown, raging with Lear-like fervour at any weak thesis statements or logical fallacies I encountered.

And then, miraculously, the baby—whom we later named Winter in gratitude for her timing—was late. Each day beyond my due date, when I had finished all my preparations, felt like a vacation, I told my doctor. I was terrified of labour and delivery, collapsing into sobs when I tried to watch birth videos. Four relaxed days after my due date, my doctor did a pelvic exam. Things were looking good, she said, and she wouldn't be surprised to see me again later that evening. Then I felt some pain of a sort I'd never encountered before. "I've just swept your membranes," she said, "That should move things along." I was flustered. As we left, my partner turned to me and asked if I was feeling all right. "She didn't ask if you wanted that done," he added. "How was that not an assault?"

I didn't know what to say. Like so many, particularly women, I was uncomfortable with the power that word would give my experience. I didn't even name the pains I felt later that afternoon "contractions," so terrified was I of the way they were sweeping me away, will I, nill I. Naming felt like my last remaining power, and I clung to it body and soul.

From the outside, I'm sure it looked like denial, a surreal refusal to accept that the process had commenced, that Pandora's box had been opened. But the truth was that I was also disproportionately terrified of reading my body incorrectly. I'd heard so many stories of first-time mothers who arrive at the hospital in panic and agony, only to be smilingly told that it was too early, and they should come back later. I couldn't bear to be a topic of laughter for my ignorance, and we lived far enough down a hole-riddled road from the hospital that I only wanted to make the journey once. By the time I was sure that these were, yes, definitely contractions, the gaps between them were smaller than the periods of breathless abstraction, and I terrified all the other occupants of the waiting room with my inability to walk down the hall to be examined.

Long before I reached this moment, pregnancy had produced an unwanted reconfiguration of my relationship to autonomy, or my control over my own bodiliness. Motherhood threatened to be a radical realignment of my rights to bodily autonomy and consent—a reformulation of my identity not as self-justifying but as secondary and instrumental to another life and other social imperatives. Pregnancy, and now motherhood, is one of those vertiginous periods—like air travel, firings, or breakups—that challenge my earnestly individualistic, not to say narcissistic, belief that the turns of my life are the product of any application of will, effort, or virtue. This false belief in personal control is bolstered by every pregnancy and parenting text, medical and literary, that I encountered ("99 Choices That You Can Make for Your Child's Health and Success!") and then mocked by others for its obsessive, narcissistic folly. Our excessive belief in individuality, this mocking strain of cultural backlash asserts, is exposed by the sheer, sublime, and terrible power of Nature (read as bodiliness) asserting its strength in our lives.

After a painful miscarriage, this pregnancy seemed to exist on a razor's edge, divorced from my choices. There was nothing I could do to prevent another cataclysm if it was coming, but if it came, the blame and criticism were certain to be laid at my feet. In this sense, pregnancy felt very much like the dread I had spent years walking through, ever since being told, at age sixteen, that a third of all women on university campuses experience assault. It was a dread not just of inevitable pain—even violence—to my body but of the moral shame that would follow. The idea that women's bodies are not their own—just vessels for the desires and needs of others—but that the blame for what happens to those bodies is wholly theirs is the cornerstone of rape culture and mother-shaming in the vast edifice of patriarchy.

I approached the due date with rising terror, with the ancients' certainty that it was inevitable as fate, but none of the Stoics' peace in facing the inexorable. Sylvia Plath, during an ill-fated or imagined pregnancy in 1959, wrote a riddle, a poem of exactly nine nine-syllable lines that weaves together the subordinating experience of gestating a child ("I'm a means, a stage, a cow in calf") with that of birthing a text ("I'm a riddle in nine syllables"). She called the poem "Metaphors," after that most literary process of transformation; metaphor is, in its most literal sense, a transfer of identity. Pregnancy is a riddle, she says, which seems to be about one thing but is, in fact, about another. It's an optical illusion that subsumes you in bodily discomforts (the shifting of your organs, the loosening of your joints, the feeling of being, as Plath puts it, "a melon strolling on two tendrils," or of having "eaten a bag of green apples") only to reveal that the process is hurtling towards erasing your body, tearing it open, and regarding it as a stage or shell for what was inside ("I've boarded the train there's no getting off"). Shift the perspective, and the pregnant body disappears, the future occluding the past and present. Teaching this to my students between snowstorms in my third trimester, they tried not to look at my belly while they dissected the connotations of Plath's diction ("yeasty," "fat," "elephant"). As they debated, I thought to myself, this poem, this idea of a pregnancy, is a hijacking—it is words taking over the body and the body fighting back. It's an Agatha Christie novel, and no one's getting off until the culprit's ready to confess. It's a Hitchcock film where the MacGuffin is my sense that I am central to my own bodily life.

In Enid Bagnold's loosely autobiographical 1938 novel, *The Squire*, a woman of means and her four children wait and wait in the humid, dreamlike final days of a pregnancy, as the baby of the family begins to feel the foundations of his tyranny crumble and an intricate politics of authority play out between the children's nurse, the midwife, and the doctor. The territory that is their battlefield is the squire's pregnant body, which is already sinking, Venice-like, into the marsh of its own importance:

> [T]he eyes of her mind lowered their lids, and she glanced with them at the embryo, impersonal, saying nothing to her, the companion. She had no tenderness for it, only the keenest expectation. It had no youth, it was old, filled with instinct. It acted like a god, as her master, directing her. She had no control over it. It had nothing to do with the born baby that was to fall with a crash from age to trembling youth, that, once born, would throw up its mastery and lie, shocked and naked, just within the gates of the world. (20)

What I dreaded most was this lack of control: the endless state of preparation, without any choice about when the pain (and change) would start. The feeling that my body was collaborating against me is what so much of midwifery tries to defuse: Remember, said my doula and the books I was reading, this is a natural process that your body is prepared for. Pain isn't, as in every other case you can remember, a sign that something is going wrong but that your body is working, working with you.

The rhetoric surrounding pain management implies that suffering was a result of an adversarial dualism, a belief that the body wars on the mind, a sort of intellectual and moral failure to move beyond Descartes. I'm sure I could manage the pain and work with it, I remember thinking, I am strong enough. But why should I? My pain is valid, but is it necessary? I became suspicious of the resemblance between celebrations of unmedicated births and Biblical arguments for why women suffer. The key thing, I thought, wasn't pain but control. For some, the raw experience of sensation in birth is control, control in the face of a titanic convulsion of the self. For others, it is the knowledge that they can and have faced such a colossal and painful task and triumphed. For me, that desperately needed trace of autonomy was fixed on the ability to silence the pain and manage my environment. I developed a horror, based largely on media representations of birth, of people shouting encouragement at me while I laboured. Having always been a contradictory sort, one who balks at the first hint of moral force, I knew that I would react badly to anything I perceived as medical bullying.

These horrors and wishes were laid out in my birth plan, a genre of text whose perfume of privilege reveals how unjust the American model of pregnancy is today. The birth plan—which pregnant parents are encouraged to craft and share with doulas, doctors, and nurses in advance of the due date—attempts to delineate every choice the parents will make in advance of it happening. This gets at the problem of consent in delivery: By the time most difficult issues arrive, the pregnant parent is sometimes so pained, exhausted, or unconscious that informed consent seems impossible. Often doulas or birth partners are delegated to act as advocates for both fetus (then baby) and pregnant patient, which can and does produce further ethical questions when the parents disagree on the best ethical course or when the parent's interests differ from the child's.

When I was pregnant, I was encouraged to write a birth plan (itself the source of some anxiety, since we didn't know what we didn't know) while also seeing scorn heaped on the very idea everywhere I looked. This is the folly of controlling, privileged mothers, I read: You can't predict birth, and you can't stage manage it. I read about the depression this fallacy of predictability created in birth parents whose labour didn't unfold according to the script. But the tone of these critiques unnerved me, along with the condemnations of mothers who schedule their C-sections to fit into packed schedules. Who do these women think they are, these think pieces seemed to ask, and why do they think they deserve control when nature will show them how powerless they truly are? At the root of these excoriations is a deep discomfort with women who think they are the agents of their own stories.

But underneath the scorn is also the reality that most parents who wield birth plans inhabit the most privileged echelons of society: we are white, affluent, urban, and enjoy access to reliable medical care from experienced professionals. And, of course, the way these plans are received reflects the privilege of the patients. The belief that one has the ability to control birth is the product of a lifetime of access to power. That this truth coexists with another is no surprise: The desire to control birth is a product of a lifetime of being told that your body (your trans body, your cis female body) is both yours to safeguard and beyond your control. All bodies deserve every thread of control they can maintain at their most vulnerable moments, but those who are most in need are least likely to have access to the modes of that autonomy (such as prenatal counselling and care, doulas, options in delivery, choice between several doctors or midwives, and birth plans).

It is in tales of birth plans gone awry that institutional violation of consent meets the feeling of being overwhelmed by bodiliness. Tina Cassidy describes her unexpected Caesarean in terms that are explicitly violent and rapacious, beginning with a cut-by-cut account of her incisions that sounds like the work of a skilled butcher: "Someone, I'm not sure who, went between my legs and up inside my body to give him an extra boost before George popped out explosively, rather like a champagne cork.... I was discharged for home feeling utterly drained, my hormones roiling, my body violently assaulted" (4). Although a great deal of the discourse of birth revels in how the delivering body turns inwards, into a sort of holistic oneness with the muscular process—parturition as, ironically enough, unity—these traumatic experiences of childbirth beyond one's control are remarkable for the way their language speaks of being partitioned, dissected, or rendered as a mere mechanical object by the rituals of the hospital and what Michel Foucault called the "medical gaze." The birthing body—associated strongly if not completely accurately with the female body—becomes a series of mechanics to be managed externally, a sort of puppet theatre, a stage for society's desires to play out like the camera carves up Marlene Dietrich's body in Laura Mulvey's theory of cinema. "Women's desire," as Mulvey says in her critique of phallocentrism, "is subjected to her image as the bearer of the bleeding wound" (7).

Allison B. Wolf and Sonya Charles, among others, point out that the medical standard for informed consent is frequently violated in the obstetrician's office and the delivery room in ways more and less severe than my experience. Among the reasons for this, they argue, citing the research of Alison Ekman Ladd, is the assumption that the process of childbirth is a de facto emergency in which medical expertise should trump bodily integrity and that "women are incompetent during labor and delivery and, thus, incapable of giving consent" (31). The stakes are especially high for patients who have experienced abuse, for whom loss of control over their own body and choices can be severely retraumatizing, as was the case for Kimberley Turbin—a rape survivor who sued her obstetrician for assault after he ignored her pleas not to proceed with an episiotomy (Grant). Judge Benny Osorio agreed with her characterization, ruling that the unconsensual intervention amounted to the legal definition of "battery."

The most extreme expression of alienation from consent in labour occurs in the last area of American society where slavery is still legal under the Constitution and where autonomy is most constrained wherever it is practiced: the prison system. Pregnant prisoners often go without adequate prenatal care, even while actively miscarrying; many experience high-risk pregnancies. Some report delivering their child alone in their cell because guards didn't believe that they were actually experiencing labour pains. Others are strip-searched while labouring before being rushed to the hospital, or shackled to the bed throughout the delivery process, or observed by armed guards as doctors and nurses do their work. Families are not permitted at the birth; sometimes they aren't even informed. Shortly afterwards, the child is taken to the prisoner's family or the foster system. Most prison systems in the United States do not provide pumping equipment or medical support to prisoners, as their milk supply painfully responds to the child's absence. Regan Clarine, imprisoned in Arizona, suffered from a Caesarian scar that kept bursting open in her cell. The guards poured sugar on it as a disinfectant (Schlanger).

Even in less extreme cases, we find echoes of the idea that bodies that give birth are not subject to the normal rules of consent, privacy, and free will. Once our daughter was born, postpartum (and later public health) nurses monitored my every biological function closely, attempting to regulate my disrupted sleep, my use of the bathroom, and, most of all, the difficult breastfeeding process. My body was constantly and unpredictably accessible to the hands and eyes of strangers. Intent on helping me, medical workers I had just met would touch my breasts unbidden to show me the correct way to engage in the natural process of breastfeeding, never happening on the same definition of correctness twice. It was not just "correct" that was hollowed out as a concept, but words like "helping" and "natural." The whole language of my postpartum life was overdetermined and coercive in its false friendliness. Eight hours into motherhood, I attempted to follow my own (natural) impulses and feed Winter when she cried. This outraged the nurse when I later confided that I found it painful: "Why would you do that without me?" she asked, adding, "Now I know I can't trust you anymore." When I tried to defer to her expertise and power by asking for advice about the pain—a beta's attempt to find safety by submitting to the dominance hierarchy of this new pack I found myself in—she waved me off in unsettling racialized terms while sweeping out the door: "It only hurts because you are so fair."

Through the haze of hormones and sleeplessness, I puzzled through my shock. This response—asserting the fragility and sensitivity of whiteness and the insensate strength of everyone excluded from that category—manages to deprive us all of solutions or solace to our pain. Black patients, especially women, routinely experience dismissal of their pain because of a belief that some races have higher pain thresholds, a falsehood that was also used to justify slavery. White patients, in turn, are only complaining of pain because they are hypersensitive to common experiences of discomfort. And whiteness is a vanishingly slippery construct, based on the relative conception of fairness that's shifted dramatically over history. In neither case is the pain regarded as real. There's no problem to be solved, no pain, discomfort, or confusion to be alleviated: instead, we needed to come to terms with the inevitability of our bodiliness. It just hurts because you are fair, or the opposite. It just hurts because you have a body, a skin, an identity. It just hurts because you gave birth. Later, the nurse returned to chide me again: "I'm worried that you are never sleeping when I come in here." I was consumed by a hypervigilance, jolting awake each time someone walked past the door, certain all my instincts were wrong and that I would be discovered in the middle of some unsanctioned act of parenthood.

I recalled these moments two years later when Serena Williams wrote a shattering account of the birth of her own first child in 2017. With access to the most expert care and greatest bodily self-knowledge in the world, the tennis champion still had her pain and unease waved off at the same point after her first birth that I had, a medical misjudgement that led to six life-threatening postpartum days of surgery and crisis. "Consider for a moment," said her husband Alexis Ohanian of that period, "that your body is one of the greatest things on this planet, and you're trapped in it" (Haskell). Williams's experience provides particular insights into why pregnancy and birth outcomes are so dramatically worse for African American women than for their white counterparts: Black babies are more than twice as likely to die in infancy, and, as a groundbreaking *New York Times* article noted, citing CDC data analyzed by the Brookings Institute, "a Black woman with an advanced degree is more likely to lose her baby than a white woman with less than an eighth-grade education" (Villarosa; Matthew, Rodrigue, and Reeves). Some researchers —among them Arline Geronimus, Richard Davis, and James Collins—have begun to articulate in recent decades how these differences are particular to the sociological environment for people of colour in the United States rather than rooted in genetic or biological causes. Geronimus theorizes that it is produced by a "weathering" effect of constant toxic stress caused by structural bigotry.

White privilege may flatter some of us as pea-tormented princesses, but it condemns us all to pain. Pregnant and postpartum bodies, gendered and racialized, are caught in a spectrum in which there is no midpoint of authority. We are too sensitive and insufficiently stoic, expected to endure pain both because of our absurd delicacy and because of our innate strength, liable to overreaction and insufficiently attentive. And patients of colour are subject to what Dána-Ain Davis calls "obstetric racism ... at the intersection of obstetric violence and medical racism" (2). Obstetric violence sees "institutional violence and violence against women coalesce during pregnancy, childbirth, and postpartum" with structural dehumanization meeting widespread misogynistic and transphobic tropes (2). Medical racism superimposes the stereotypes of prejudice on the patient, including the idea that Black women's bodies are "medical superbodies ... worthy enough for labor and experimentation" and impervious to pain and weakness while "the woman herself is not worthy of being treated humanely" (2). Thus, these bodies are asked to step into scripts that prejudice and projection have wrought and sociological scenes and roles that don't fit them but seem destined for them by race, gender, and medical status.

In 2019, for instance, the Tl'etinqox band in British Columbia battled provincial authorities to reunite a young family. The first-time parents were separated from their child when a neglect report was made ninety minutes into the baby's life. Social workers, arguing with the family in the hospital room, pointed to the mother's vagueness as support for the action; the father replied that she was still under the effects of the sedation she'd been given for her emergency C-section just hours before.

This is not an unprecedented story in contemporary Canada. In Manitoba, where inexperience with parenting, poverty, or time spent in women's shelters after leaving an abuser can be cited as reasons to take infants into the foster system, Indigenous parents report that they are forced to avoid hospitals when the time comes to deliver, giving birth in secret because children are so often taken from maternity wards (Edwards).

Yet the medical system within which we all operate errs on the side of personalizing responsibility to the patient—and especially to the patient of colour—rather than acknowledging the inescapable structural pressure of this weathering and scrutiny. Through a backformation of bigoted logic, poor medical outcomes are assumed by medical and governmental authorities to be the result of negligence and abuse (an umbrella term that perilously encompasses drinking, drug use, unemployment, poverty, as well as inconsistent access to shelter or food) even when there is no evidence to support that assumption. Poor health outcomes for African American women and their infants were assumed to be the result of higher poverty and substance abuse— always coded as the moral responsibility of the individual. Data emerged, however, showing Black women were less likely to consume alcohol or tobacco while pregnant and that none of the individual actions that had been suggested as paternalistic solutions—for example, prenatal education, education, avoidance of teen pregnancy, and diet—correlated to the negative outcomes. There is no personal choice a pregnant person can make to affect these outcomes, yet the solutions suggested turn the problem back on the individual in ways that are both blaming and shaming. Stress is known to be toxic for pregnant people and their fetuses, but the experience of reproduction is one of anxious scrutiny and surveillance in both the United States and Canada, based largely on the underlying assumption that the pregnant body is always already unruly, disobedient, and untrustworthy.

The twenty-four hours surrounding the birth of my first child—from the moment when my doctor painfully intervened, without asking, in my reproductive organs to the moment when I finally drifted off for a few minutes with a tiny baby in my arms I was frightened to feed— revealed several horrifying truths to me. We conceive of the maternal body as a medical object to be monitored and controlled while also maintaining that the transition into motherhood is a natural and instinctive process in which the suffering or befuddled body is denied and obscured. Women (particularly women of colour and Indigenous women, and to an even greater degree trans and nonbinary people) who are pregnant, miscarrying, grieving, recuperating, nursing, or simply parenting are caught in a crux of violation between a pathological view of their bodies and a denial of the pains and confusions that accompany the role. Institutional medicine and social practice have placed pregnant and postpartum bodies in this paradoxical trap, with violation and anxiety on every side. How do we navigate the unique role of pregnancy and its aftermath as mostly healthy but also painful processes? By not denying the autonomy of choice to patients who already feel subordinated to other lives or our own runaway bodies.

Works Cited

Bagnold, Enid. *The Squire.* Persephone, 2013.

Cassidy, Tina. *Birth: The Surprising History of How We Are Born.* Grove Atlantic, 2006.

Davis, Dána-Ain. "Obstetric Racism: the Politics of Pregnancy, Labor, and Birthing." *Medical Anthropology*, 2018, vol. 38, no. 3, pp. 1-14.

Edwards, Kyle. "Fighting Foster Care." *Macleans*, 9 Jan. 2018, www. macleans.ca/first-nations-fighting-foster-care/. Accessed 3 Aug. 2019.

Foucault, Michel. *The Birth of the Clinic: An Archaeology of Medical Perception.* Vintage Books, 1975.

Geronimus, E. T. "The Weathering Hypothesis and the Health of African-American Women and Infants: Evidence and Speculations." *Ethnicity and Disease*, vol. 2, no. 2, 1992, pp. 207-21.

Grant, Rebecca. "Doctors Who Ignore Consent Are Traumatizing Women during Childbirth." *Quartz*, 5 Dec. 2017, www. qz. com/1146836/doctors-who-ignore-consent-are-traumatizing-women-during-childbirth/. Accessed 30 Jun. 2019.

Haskell, Rob. "Serena Williams on Motherhood, Marriage, and Making Her Comeback." *Vogue*, 10 Jan. 2018, www.vogue.com/ article/serena-williams-vogue-cover-interview-february-2018. Accessed 5 Apr. 2021.

Ladd, Rosalind Ekman. "Women in Labor: Some Issues About Informed Consent." *Hypatia*, vol. 4, no. 3, 1989, 37-45.

Matthew, Dana Bowen, Edward Rodrigue, and Richard V. Reeves. "Time for Justice: Tackling Racial Inequalities in Health and Housing." *Brookings*, 9 Oct. 2016, www.brookings.edu/research/time-for-justice-tackling-race-inequalities-in-health-and-housing/. Accessed 2 Aug. 2019.

Mulvey, Laura. "Visual Pleasure and Narrative Cinema." *Screen*, vol. 16, issue 3, 1975, pp. 6-18.

Plath, Sylvia. *The Collected Poems*. Harper Perennial, 2018.

Schlanger, Zoë. "What It's Like to Give Birth in a U.S. Prison." *Quartz*, 6 Apr. 2019. www.qz.com/1587102/what-its-like-to-give-birth-in-a-us-prison/. Accessed 15 Jul. 2019.

Villarosa, Linda. "Why America's Mothers and Babies are in a Life or Death Crisis." *The New York Times*, 11 Apr. 2018, www.nytimes.com/2018/04/11/magazine/black-mothers-babies-death-maternal-mortality.html. Accessed 23 Mar. 2021.

Wolf, Alison B. and Sonya Charles. "Childbirth is not an Emergency: Informed Consent in Labor and Delivery." *IJFAB*, vol. 11, no. 1, 2018, 23-43.

Chapter 5

Dr. Mom Meets the Brain Surgeon

Sharon McCutcheon

Before my medical training began, my husband, Greg, and I lived in a small rural community in southern New Brunswick. As a mother with three young children, I knew there would be many challenges in reaching my goal to become a doctor, some of them almost insurmountable at times, because I was a mother. In 1992, I filled out the application to medical school on an old-fashioned typewriter at my kitchen table, while our three young children played noisily in the next room. We lived in a small, one-level house and there was nowhere else for the kids to play. A friend who was visiting that day looked at the chaos of my home with raised eyebrows and asked how I ever hoped to complete the application, let alone attend medical school. At the time, I really wasn't sure. Writing the forms was minor in comparison to what was ahead, and my children would be there throughout the journey.

No one was more shocked than I was when I was granted an interview. I had decided that hiding the fact that I had children was irrelevant. In a room with three interviewers, we discussed many topics concerning my previous achievements at university, my volunteer work, and my employment over the past few years. We talked of coping with stress and the gruelling pace of a medical career. When I mentioned that my husband and three children would be a support to me and keep me grounded, looks were exchanged, and I was questioned about how I expected to cope with being a mother in medical school. At the time, perhaps it was reasonable to doubt my ability to balance motherhood and a medical career, but I wondered if the same concerns were ever brought up with the male candidates who were married with children.

I felt that I had performed well in the interview and the group exercises, but the interviewer's questions caused a lot of personal doubt as to whether I could really do it. I told myself that the kids would be at school during the weekdays, that I could study at night, and that my husband would step in to help. I think I underestimated the time that would be spent on helping my kids with homework, family stresses, or even the housework that would now fall mostly to Greg. Luckily, he was supportive and agreed to leave his job to make the move half way across the country that would change our lives forever.

After receiving my acceptance letter, our next obstacle was a lack of financial stability. We experienced a lot of negativity and concern from well-meaning family and friends. Instead of the excited and supportive reaction I expected with the news of my acceptance to medical school and the opportunity to fulfill my dream of becoming a doctor, I encountered disapproval and doubt. My father was less than enthusiastic, saying, "You have a husband and three kids to think about now, and your head is still in the clouds." I wondered if I had been a son instead of a daughter whether it would have been different and more acceptable.

People were aghast that I was actually planning to do this. Instead of praise and encouragement, my news was met with disbelief that I would even consider it, since I had kids. Another mother in the community said to me, "I could never do what you are doing." Thinking that she was complimenting me on my intellectual abilities, I was shocked when she added: "I love my children too much." Although I was still determined to make it all work, I began to feel incredible guilt. I told myself that my kids would see me as a role model who would inspire them to reach for their own dreams later. Still, I wondered if everyone thought I was putting my own goals ahead of my children.

After the stressful experience of moving to another province where we knew no one, I entered McMaster Medical School in Hamilton, Ontario, when my kids were six, eight, and ten. As the only mother of three in a class of one hundred medical students, the challenges I faced started early in the process of becoming a doctor. From the first few days, I found that I was considered the oddity in the group. Even though it was probably what I most needed to feel a part of my class, attending social events often proved impossible, as I already had little time with my children and our budget was low. While I was heading home to make supper, help with homework and get the kids ready for bed, I knew that my classmates were often heading home to a quiet apartment where they could study.

Our children made friends quickly in our multicultural neighbourhood, and I was relieved to think that they would have many positive experiences due to the move. As a mother in medical school, I tried to provide activities that would ensure that we had some quality time together. We hiked on the nearby trails and spent time with neighbours, who treated us like family for the whole five years of my training. An elderly couple who lived on the same street became like surrogate grandparents to our children, while I was devoting more time to my studies.

I was grateful for the support from a few classmates, both male and female. Some brought treats for the kids and helped in many ways. The majority of the other students were unaware of the struggles we faced and likely only realized what it was like after they had kids of their own, later in their careers. This was not surprising to me as I did not expect them to understand my situation in the middle of their own unique experiences.

A girl in my class was upset one morning when her cat went missing. I tried to console her, saying, "Your cat will likely be waiting on your doorstep when you get home." She looked at me and said, "Do you even know where your kids are?" The comment was said spontaneously, without thought, but reminded me of the judgments that people make when mothers choose untraditional careers. Although we like to think that many things have changed, there is a still a stigma, and it is sometimes other women who have negative feelings about balancing medicine and motherhood.

The support from the medical faculty was better than I had expected, and I think this relates to the fact that by the time physicians are established in their careers, they have likely already started their families. One day the school called to tell me that Julie, our youngest daughter, was sick. I approached my supervising physician to explain and ask if I could leave to pick her up. Fearing a negative reaction, I was surprised when he put his hand on my shoulder and said, with kindness, "Of course you can go. I have five children. Medicine will always be here, but your children will only be little for such a short time."

While on-call and spending nights at the hospital, I think that initially I had an advantage, as I had no illusions about fatigue and sleepless nights. I was a mother; it was already a part of my life. However, when I added the caregiving tasks when my own children were ill, nights at the hospital and studying long past midnight became detrimental to my own physical and mental health. I was never able to go home to a quiet place and relax on the couch. As much as my spouse was supportive in helping out, he had his limits too and my exhaustion forced me to delegate more and more of our children's needs to him. While his role became a combination of mother and father at times, my role as a mother amidst the overwhelming pace of my medical studies often seemed exhausting and impossible as I struggled to become "Doctor Mom."

Greg rose to the challenge, but my medical training sometimes added considerable stress to our relationship, as more and more of my time was spent away from our children. I think I underestimated how much energy it took for him to hold down the fort through the many times that I was not available, physically or emotionally, due to my medical responsibilities. He was expected to understand the toll it took on my psychological health and my capabilities as a mother, especially when I struggled with the new experiences of witnessing pain, suffering, death and dying on a daily basis. In addition, anxiety, fatigue, and later depression started to become more of an issue, as a result of trying to balance my two roles. Male and female physicians have the same stressors during their careers, but mothers who are doctors often carry an added burden of increased caregiving, household tasks, and guilt, even with a supportive spouse.

Early in my career, my children were forced to learn independence and self-reliance, and they often struggled with my absence as a parent. Unknowingly, I handed some of my stress over to my kids, oblivious that they were literally going through medical school too, as I became "Doctor Mom." I didn't notice the irony that even this title still put doctor ahead of being a mother. My husband was also learning about medicine through his daily conversations with me, although he received no diploma at the end of my studies. There were many unmet expectations on both sides in our relationship, and many times I heard my kids express, "Why can't you just be a normal mom?"

When our youngest daughter was a teenager, she was sometimes angry when I was unable to be there for her due to the responsibilities of my career. One day, she left me a note that said: "I know your job is stressful and important, but I'm your daughter, and I am important, too. Sometimes I think that I am still that little girl who thinks her mother is there solely to take care of her. And for that, I am sorry." I was devastated to think that she felt the need to apologize for needing me.

As much as I always wanted to put my children first, sometimes it was impossible. As a doctor, I was focused on the concerns of my patients, and by the end of the day, it was not an easy transition from being a doctor at a busy clinic to being a wife and mother. I was often distracted and irritable with Greg and the kids. I felt that I had little control over the hours I spent away from them and the constant switching of roles that I had to maintain. I think this is true of everyone in the medical field but even more so for mothers.

I frequently taught medical students and residents in my practice. One resident had a small baby and was still breastfeeding. I wanted to make sure she felt supported, so I asked about priorities during the rotation. Thinking that I was asking about her commitment to her medical training, she assured me that she would not neglect her education as she had help from her spouse. At that moment, I realized that we had not progressed very far in supporting women in medicine. I told her that she would not have to express milk in the bathroom or hide the fact that she was a new mother, and if her child was sick, her child came first. I hoped that this discussion was a catalyst for change, at least for her.

After fifteen years as a busy family doctor, I thought I had become somewhat accustomed to the stress of medicine, and my children were now grown and independent. Then in 2011, I had a CT scan, which was done to diagnose a sinus problem. With Greg still in the waiting room, the radiologist called me in to see the results that revealed a large brain tumour. Pointing to the very visible tumour, the radiologist commented: "Sharon, you likely need surgery pretty quickly as there is some midline shift." I felt like I was looking at someone else's scan, as I was still in the role of doctor. "Looks like a meningioma, most likely benign," he said. It was still a life-changing diagnosis for me. It also reminded me of my own vulnerability, of how hard I had worked to become a doctor, while balancing motherhood with my career. Now, after all of the sacrifices, I was diagnosed with a brain tumour.

Usually, a patient would leave the CT department and have an appointment later with their own doctor, who would prepare to give them bad news, which would generally be in the presence of a family member who could offer support. Instead, I told my husband the news in the elevator, as the radiologist had already set up an expedited appointment upstairs to see a neurosurgeon. Instead of going out for pizza as planned, we headed up for the appointment. An MRI with an angiogram was scheduled for that evening. My family doctor was not informed until later. Although I appreciated the professional courtesy and the speed and efficiency of this, I was numb from the shock of the news. All I could think about was how it would affect my family and my patients. Telling my kids would be the next hurdle. I realized that this was one more stress that I would hand over to them. To my colleagues, it seemed that it was just another day at the office. To me, it was a bombshell. When I arrived to speak to the neurosurgeon, who was also a colleague, he poked his head out of his office door and said, "Hello Sharon, are you okay?" I wanted to say, "Obviously not, as apparently, I have a brain tumour." Still in my professional role, I smiled and said, "Yes. I'm okay." Then he asked if I minded if he finished a dictation before speaking with us. His secretary, who wanted to leave at the end of a long day, handed me a consent form for brain surgery to complete while I waited. This was all done with kindness and respect, but I wondered if the fact that I was a doctor changed the appointment slightly. Suddenly, he had become the esteemed neurosurgeon and I the vulnerable patient.

I had great difficulty with the lack of control that a medical crisis brought. Doctors are the ones who order the tests, write the prescriptions, and decide on a treatment plan. When I was diagnosed, it was a much different experience than I believe most patients have with a critical health issue. Sometimes I was treated as a doctor first and as a patient second. Sadly, my role as a mother seemed to come last, while my family struggled to cope with my diagnosis.

Over the years, my career had already added tremendous tension to our family life and now this new diagnosis plunged us into chaos. Yet I was expected to plan for the care of my patients, who were suddenly without a doctor, as well as trying to spend more time with my husband and kids. I learned that my responsibilities would either follow me or they would be waiting there in the shadows until I returned. I began to understand that my career was more stressful than the brain tumour. I was also expected to intuitively know how to cope with the strain of my own health crisis while coping with my kids' reactions and my career at the same time.

After the diagnosis, I continued to work in the office for several days to wrap up details and try to entice a locum to take over my clinic. Between patients, my partner came in to ask what my plans were. So overwhelmed with the whole situation, I sat with my head in my hands and cried while the resident that I was supervising handed me Kleenex. Then I pulled myself together and went in to see the next patient, trying to look composed and professional. My daughter called me a few minutes later and said, "Mom, please come home. We need you, too." As a physician, I never felt that I could just walk away from my medical responsibilities and deal with the profound stress the brain tumour was causing us as a family.

In the time leading up to the surgery, I requested that my family come in with me to ask the neurosurgeon some questions about potential adverse events. It was extremely important to me that the neurosurgeon see me as a wife, a mother, and a grandmother and not just as a colleague. I thought that it was important that he understood how all of this would affect my children as well as how it affected me as a mother.

During the surreal experience of brain surgery, I was reminded of the years in a medical career that had changed my experience as a mother when my oldest daughter brought my two grandchildren, a baby and a toddler, into Neuro ICU. I agonized over the thought that there was a chance that I could also be robbed of the full experience of being a grandmother, if I was not around to see my little grandkids grow up.

I was readmitted twelve days after discharge for a second surgery to remove a piece of my skull due to complications of a bone flap infection. Several weeks of IV antibiotics followed and then a third surgery scheduled a few months later for insertion of an acrylic plate. Between the second and third surgeries, I was told that I could return to work and that my patients needed me. At the time, I felt that my kids and my husband needed me even more. My family had been in crisis mode for months, and I was expected to put their needs aside again so I could go back to work. My children were thrust into the role of looking after me, even though I wanted to be the mother who provided for their needs during a family crisis.

I returned to work within six months, after three surgeries. There was never a question that I might not be ready to return to a busy medical practice. Despite having brain surgery with complications, I was told that I was doing well enough that I could return to work "whenever I wanted." Colleagues were encouraging me to return as soon as possible, and I felt incredible guilt that I did not feel cognitively safe or emotionally ready to return. Like being a mother, I felt that being a doctor meant putting the needs of others ahead of my own. Despite my misgivings, I gave in to the pressure and continued to practice for another six years, until worsening seizures led to the closure of my practice.

Balancing motherhood with a medical career was a constant struggle. This was only fully realized after my retirement, when I looked back over the time spent on my career, which had led to diminished time with my children. Becoming a grandmother was a blessing, especially since I was able to spend more time with family after I stopped working due to my own medical issues.

I often leaned heavily on my family for support, and my children had to adapt to having a mother who was not always available. At times, it meant putting the needs of my patients over the needs of my kids, often missing family events or activities when I was working late or on call. Most importantly, my role as a doctor added significant stress to our family life. Yet being a mother enhanced my medical career, as I felt more of an affinity for mothers in my practice. Motherhood was a place of common ground: it gave me a better understanding of issues my female patients faced, such as breastfeeding, the stress of parenting, and balancing a career with motherhood.

My intersecting roles of mother and doctor were challenged when I myself became the patient. Balancing both of these caregiving roles became impossible to maintain after I became the one who needed care. The role of doctor as patient illustrates the many unique challenges doctors face in navigating personal healthcare experiences. For me, becoming a patient highlighted the lack of support for physicians with a medical crisis. This lack of support is all the more salient when the patient is both physician and mother. As mothers, we are conditioned to care for our babies, and in a medical career, we are conditioned to care for our patients, yet we find it so difficult to put ourselves first and accept care when we need it.

Surviving a brain tumour during my medical career highlights my perception that my experiences during my diagnosis, surgeries, and recovery were even more overwhelming, as I was still expected to balance the responsibilities of my medical career with my role as a mother during my own health crisis. Mothers in medicine become resilient out of necessity, but we still need additional support to successfully balance our roles as caregivers, especially when we also become the patient.

Chapter 6

"Usually the Mother": Dilation and the Medical Management of Intersex Children

Celeste E. Orr and Amanda D. Watson

The routine medical genital mutilation of people with intersex variations—particularly infants, children, and adolescents—is well documented (Davis; Dreger; Preves; Karkazis; Morland; Koyama; Kessler; Cornwall; Greenberg; Chase; Orr). However, too few studies (Karkazis) critically examine or theorize intersex people's parents' experiences with medical professionals and the role that parents play in treating their pathologized intersex children. The fact that analyses are scant is noteworthy: Intersex people often reference their mothers when recounting experiences of medical trauma (Wall; Inter; "Not a Girl"; Pagonis, "9 Damaging Lies"). Moreover, vaginal dilation, one of the so-called treatments prescribed by medical professionals, often falls to the mother. Hence, this chapter asks the following: Why are mothers uniquely involved in their intersex children's treatment and what are the implications of their involvement?

Dilation with a medical dildolike device is intended to ensure the sociomedically assigned girl child's "shallow" or surgically constructed vagina does not close off: "When they surgically 'create' a vagina on a child, the parent—usually the mother—is required to 'dilate' the vagina with hard instruments every day for months in order to ensure that the vagina won't close off again" (Koyama 2). Many intersex studies scholars and activists refer to this practice as "ritualistic" (2), "institutionalized" (Arana 31), as well as sexual abuse of intersex children (Orr, *Exorcizing Intersex* 131; Astorino; Alexander; Tosh; Guillot, Bauer, and Truffer). Mothers understandably following doctors' orders; thus, they become complicit in sexual abuse, which strains or destroys their child-mother relationship (Karkazis).

Mothers' involvement in dilating their assigned-girl intersex children is understudied. Drawing from intersex, feminist, and motherhood studies, as well as attending to mothers' involvement in dilation, we posit that mothers are compelled to perform this abusive, traumatizing act because (1) mothers are disproportionately expected to make decisions regarding the care of their children (Apple, "Perfect Motherhood"; Baillargeon) and (2) dilation will not be read as sexual abuse if performed by the mother rather than the father due to gender norms. Given that childcare tasks are gendered, particularly when children are young, well-intentioned mothers come to perform dilation on their intersex children and, thus, cause harm to their children and familial relationships.

This chapter also considers how the intersex rights movement might inspire new ways of thinking about care, pathologization, disability, maternal responsibility, and violence. The mutilating and sexually abusive practice of dilation, whereby mothers become instruments of the medical establishment, echoes the familiar social expectation of mothers to pursue the direction of medical experts for their own good and the good of their families. As both Amanda Watson (*Juggling Mother*) and Ana Villalobos have shown, mothers' efforts to secure wellbeing for their children and families can come at the expense of their own wellbeing and can enforce status quo hierarchies of power. The accounts of intersex people illustrate that mothers are positioned to fail as they mediate between their children and medical professionals, which calls into question the role of parents as they advocate for pathologized intersex children.

Undermining Compulsory Dyadism

Intersex is a general term used to describe people with inborn physical, hormonal, or genetic traits that defy the Western sociomedical male-female sex binary. As such, "there is no single 'intersex body'; [intersex] encompasses a wide variety of conditions" or embodiments "that do not have anything in common except that they are deemed 'abnormal' by the society. What makes intersex people similar is their experiences of medicalization, not biology" ("Intersex FAQ"). In Celeste E. Orr's terms, intersex people undermine "compulsory dyadism"—the instituted cultural mandate that people cannot have intersex traits and must embody and reaffirm the male-female sex dyad (*Exorcizing Intersex* 37-49). As a result, intersex is pathologized and rendered disordered, disabled, or diseased (Davis, *Contesting Intersex*; Viloria; Holmes; Orr, *Exorcising Intersex*). The logic of pathologization then necessitates remedial medical interventions. In fact, intersex variations are often framed as medical "emergencies," despite the fact that intersex traits rarely, if ever, cause medical problems or illnesses (Karkazis 96; Davis *Contesting Intersex*). In a horribly ironic twist, as Orr argues elsewhere, said medical interventions constitute "curative violence" (Kim 10; Orr, *Exorcizing Intersex* 54). As Eunjung Kim argues, "Curative violence occurs when cure is what actually frames the presence of disability as a problem and ends up destroying the subject in the curative process" (14). Under the current medical model, what is deemed disabled or disordered requires a medical response or cure. Intersex people typically experience medicalization and curative, violent procedures intended to reorder sex, but they ultimately cause profound harm.

Intersex people are routinely subjected to nonconsensual, medically unnecessary surgeries (intersex genital mutilation [IGM]), hormone replacement therapy (HRT), vaginal dilation, and/or consistent medical surveillance to ensure their body-minds[1] better approximate compulsory dyadism. These so-called curative procedures typically result in many short- and long-term consequences, such as the following: infection, genital pain, (painful) scarring, loss of sexual sensation, the need for urinary assistive devices, anesthetic neurotoxicity, incontinence, anxiety, fear of intimacy, depression, PTSD, and suicidal ideation. Indeed, these consequences constitute body-mind disabilities (Orr, *Exorcizing Intersex* 76).

Many intersex people and intersex studies scholars note how various oppressive systems—interphobia, heterosexism, phallogocentrism, queerphobia, as well as compulsory dyadism, heterosexuality, and able-bodiedness—work together to justify curative violence. In many intersex people's testimonies about curative violence, they describe their parents', often their mothers', involvement in and navigation of the medical system that seeks to cure them. Even so, the experiences of intersex people's parents and their relationship to medical management are not well theorized or understood.

Parents' Relationships to Intersex Medical Management

Historically, and still to varying degrees today, parents are encouraged "never to discuss the [intersex] diagnosis with others or the child, thus instilling extraordinary shame in parents (and hence the child)" (Karkazis 2; also see Davis, "Interview"). Given that intersex is stigmatized, literally and figuratively erased, and pathologized, parents understandably internalize interphobic shame. It is unsurprising that mothers—who, if they are birthing people, have pregnancy and postpartum experiences mediated by professions of paediatrics and obstetrics and whose childcare responsibilities are most likely to involve interaction with medical professionals—receive and process the stigmatization of their children uniquely. When Vincent Guillot was born with intersex traits, for example, his mother was told that "she had given birth to a monster" ("Not a Girl"). Vincent's mother was thrust into the realm of interphobic judgment and shame from a powerful institution immediately upon giving birth.

Given that medical professionals expect the mothers of intersex children to internalize status quo interphobia and become complicit in medical intervention and the erasure of diagnoses and medical procedures in raising their intersex children, many are concerned with gender nonconforming behaviour in their children (Karkazis 196). Mothering duties concerning culturally appropriate gender rearing are complicated when their child is intersex; they are consistently called to view their child as at a pathological risk of being outcast by their peers and becoming queer, trans, or gender nonconforming. Consequently, as outlined below, many intersex people speak of strained relationships with their mothers.

Mothers understandably desire their children to live full, happy lives. Medical professionals teach mothers that their intersex children will not be able to live such lives without curative medical procedures and concerted rearing as exclusively heterosexual boys or girls (Holmes; Davis, *Contesting Intersex*; Karkazis). Many mothers, therefore, agree to curative violence without fully understanding the violence until much later. For example, Debbie Hartman, mother to Kelli, an intersex child, describes being told that forgoing medical intervention would cause Kelli unbearable distress (qtd. in Arana). Hartman was not provided with enough information to make a fully informed decision about surgery; when she asked to speak with other parents of intersex children or intersex people themselves, she was, like many others, falsely told "there is no one" (Hartman qtd. in Arana 48). Due to being misinformed and understandably believing Kelli's doctors had Kelli's best interests in mind, Hartman assumed surgery was the right choice and agreed to the procedure. Hartman realized later that Kelli had "endured unnecessary pain, confusion and severe emotional and physical scarring" (qtd. in Arana 48). Hartman further recounts: "My child has tried to commit suicide twice in her 10 little years because she says she hates her body.... She constantly asks me why they ... cut up her genitals" (qtd. in Arana 48). Hartman reports Kelli stating: "They thought I was no good, Mom" (qtd. in Arana 48). How complicated for a child to resent the mutilation allowed by their mother and for a mother to realize that unwanted violence and ongoing body-mind crisis ruined her efforts to advocate for her child's wellbeing and social inclusion.

Collaborating with Enemies

Intersex people primarily blame medical professionals, the medical industrial complex, and pathologizing and discriminatory ideologies for the trauma and body-mind disabilities they acquire via curative violence. However, many intersex people's stories highlight the role of parents, particularly mothers for facilitating their medical interventions, for failing to disclose medical information, and for reinforcing interphobia and queerphobia in their childrearing practices. For instance, Jean Butler recounts the following:

> The cue I got early on from my mother was, "Don't talk about this." When I was about six and my older sister was eight, she and I just had our baths, and we were playing naked on the bed and giving ourselves a genital examination. I counted that she has three holes and I only had two. We thought this was uproariously funny, and I went running over to my mother saying, "Susan has three holes, and I only have two," and my mother just said to me sternly, "Get to bed." That was it. We never discussed it again....

I had a couple of other experiences with my mom ... and finally I just closed up. I had the feeling that there was no recognition....
I tried once to bring up my surgery with my mother and she said, "Your doctors assure me that you're just perfectly normal after your surgery, there's nothing wrong at all." That was basically her attitude: surgery was fine and there's no problem. I think she didn't feel comfortable going into it, and as a result I didn't either. (qtd. in Karkazis 220)

According to Katrina Karkazis, these moments in Butler's life "curtailed all openness in her family about her diagnosis" (220). But it is clear in Butler's testimony that her mother is at the helm of the silence and lack of recognition that characterized Butler's childhood experiences of interphobia and shame.

Likewise, Sean Saifa M. Wall—an intersex activist, writer, and artist, who was sociomedically assigned female but identifies as a Black intersex man—elaborates on his experiences with his mother amid navigating the treacherous waters of curative violence and his gender:

The pain that I felt following the surgery was perhaps the worst pain that I have experienced in my entire life. After surgery, my pediatrician prescribed estrogen and Provera as a hormonal replacement regimen. Fatty deposits changed the shape and contours of my face. Once robust and chiseled thighs now harbored cellulite. The beginnings of facial hair and prominent body hair became wispy and nonexistent.... At no point did anyone ask me what I wanted to do with my body. I actually missed the effects of my natural testosterone such as a deepening voice, increased hair and muscle mass; when I asked if I could take both testosterone and estrogen after surgery, my mother remarked, "You would look too weird." The hormone therapy was coupled with intense social conditioning ... the social conditioning for young women raised with AIS [androgen insensitivity syndrome] is suffocating. When doctors prescribed hormones for me to take, my mother constantly reminded me how "beautiful" the little yellow pills would make me. (Wall, 118)

In her rejection of Wall's request for testosterone, his mother signals a desire for cisheteronormative presentation and her own fear driving this particular intervention: He will be excluded, she will be judged negatively, or both.

In addition to surgeries and HRT, many intersex children are subjected to consistent, gratuitous medical monitoring, genital displays, and examinations to ensure they are developing properly according to heteronormative and dyadic ideas about sex and gender. Laura Inter (pseud.) was subjected to such examinations:

> From the time I turned one, I was subjected to genital exam-
> inations twice a year, during which the endocrinologist would
> touch my genitals and look to see how they were developing.
> These unnecessary and intrusive examinations had a profound
> effect on me. As a young child, I did not understand why I had to
> lower my pants in front of a stranger—the endocrinologist—and
> let him touch me. The fact that my mother was present, and
> approved of this was something that made me feel completely
> helpless.... I found it confusing, and terribly uncomfortable, and
> I just felt it wasn't right.... I grew up with a feeling of being
> "inadequate," of having a sense that something was wrong with
> me, though I didn't know exactly what. These exams lasted until
> I was about 12 years old. Years later.... I realized how much those
> displays had affected me emotionally. (Inter 95)

For Inter, their mother's approval of these invasive, humiliating examinations left them bewildered, scared, and betrayed. Michel Reiter reports feeling similarly: "I had about 200 examinations in my life. I didn't want these examinations, but my mother took me to them. I didn't trust her. I saw her collaborating with my enemies" (qtd. in Lahood). As guardians and caregivers, mothers' advocacy sadly fails to defend the needs or autonomy of their children.

As a child, Pidgeon Pagonis was told they were born with cancer to avoid telling them they were born with intersex traits. Although there is no definitive evidence that intersex traits will develop cancer at a quicker rate than endosex (nonintersex) traits (Carpenter; Orr, *Exorcising Intersex* 118-20), Pagonis's parents were told their child would develop cancer, and they were advised to tell Pagonis they were born with cancer. Pagonis writes:

> One of the first lies my mother told me was that I was born with
> cancerous ovaries and that they were removed in a life-saving
> post-birth operation. You [doctors] instructed my parents to tell

me this made-up story, and it became a root in my development. When I began asking questions about why I couldn't get a period or have biological children, you told my mother to just stick to the cancer story—and she did.... You didn't tell my parents the same lie. Instead of telling them I was born with cancer, you hyped the risk that my "underdeveloped ovaries" which you decisively referred to as "gonads"—and really were my undescended testes—would likely develop cancer if left intact. You noted in the records after my gonadectomy that the tissue samples came back negative and "no term other than gonad was used." This manipulative tactic meant to induce willingness in scared parents is a byproduct of a culture that insists, sometimes by force, that humans only come in two polar opposite varieties. Instead of removing my undescended testes and causing a life-long dependency on hormone replacement therapy ... you could have instead been honest with us and offered to monitor them annually for signs of cancer.... These types of decisions about our bodies belong to us and never to you. (Pagonis, "9 Damaging Lies"; also see Pagonis, "The Son They Never Had"; Davis, "Interview").

Though Pagonis mentions both of their parents, it seems clear in their repeated mention of the mother that their mother stands out as both the target of interphobic medical propaganda as well as the one responsible for propagating lies. Since mothers are disproportionately responsible for the emotional management work of childrearing (Watson, "Quelling Anxiety"), it seems inevitable that the mother would be caught in this position and also maybe especially upsetting for a child if she is supposed to be the one ultimately protecting her child's best interests.

Although mothers (and parents in general) are not blameless, attending to the fact that intersex people's stories mention mothers brings to light how mothers are disproportionally responsible for the childrearing labour of gender socialization, communicating with medical providers, and attending doctor appointments. Mothers then are typically the ones who agree to, witness, and assist in curative violence, or, in Reiter's terms, collaborate with enemies. Analyzing the specific intervention of vaginal dilation through feminist studies of motherwork helps us further unpack mothers' involvement in the medical process, unfolding stories of misogyny, sexism, violence, and abuse of power by caregivers.

In the case of curative violence against intersex people, mothers are instructed to perform a cruel violation that undermines their obligation to advocate for their children and the unfair expectation that mothers put the needs of their children before themselves (Villalobos). The responsible mother follows doctor's orders, advocates for her children, and is responsible for her children's wellbeing. In this context, the mother of an intersex child is positioned to fail. In following doctors' directions—likely at a time in the development of her identity as a mother-advocate when things seem particularly uncertain and fraught—she enacts a prolonged, sexually invasive procedure on her child. In this context, it is not hard to imagine how mothers might find relief of their internal tensions by relying on the interphobic messages of established medical practice and the promise of greater health outcomes and social inclusion for their children. Indeed, it would be surprising if mothers performed vaginal dilation practices without relying on and internalizing interphobia to justify their actions to themselves.

Vaginal Dilation

Vaginal dilation, one of many forms of curative violence some intersex people are subjected to, involves dilating assigned girl children and adolescents with hard dildolike instruments whose vaginas are deemed too small or shallow to accommodate a prospective normal-sized penis. Evidently shaped by the intersecting logics of compulsory dyadism, heterosexuality, and able-bodiedness, medical dilators are employed to (1) nonsurgically deepen vaginas that do not have a uterus or cervix or (2) maintain or additionally stretch vaginas surgically constructed by vaginoplasties. In Kira Triea's terms, procedures like dilation are performed to "make the hermaphrodite fuckable" to prospective adult cishet men (143).

Many intersex people have undergone countless dilation procedures over months or years. The disabling violence and negative consequences of both vaginoplasties and dilation are profound. Vaginoplasties "can cause infertility ... the constructed vagina can smell like a bowel; it can necessitate constant use of sanitary napkins; it frequently requires repeated surgical revisions; and it is usually created or deepened for the expressed goal of accommodating a penis, rather than for the satisfaction of the patients" (Arana 21; also see Hillman in Clearway). And dilation during genital examinations "is often painful and humiliating" (Arana 21). Gina Wilson confirms: "The psychological effects" of "therapeutically" dilating or "penetrating" children in this manner are extremely damaging. The intersex children's sexual pleasure as well as ability to orgasm, reproduce, and move through the world comfortably are sacrificed to maintain numerous discriminatory ideologies, uphold compulsory modes of being, and privilege cishet men's (potential) sexual pleasure. These children's body-minds and sexual agency are not treated or conceptualized as their own. Instead, medical professionals (and mothers) manage them.

Claudia Astorino explains that dilation occurs to ensure that the vagina is "long enough to fit a penis inside of it" and documents her own experiences:

> I had a dilation procedure performed for almost every exam I had with intersex doctors from the time I was 8 until I was 16, so that they could check how long my vagina was as I grew. I absolutely hated these procedures. I mean, imagine a man as old as your father or your grandfather, who you don't know, inserting a medical dildo into you each time you saw him, knowing that you can't question the doctor's orders and just accept that you have to undergo these uncomfortable procedures for your health. Imagine a decade or so later, realizing that these procedures did nothing to track your health, and have everything to with grown men feeling good about the fact that you could fuck some dude someday like a "normal girl." That all those traumatizing procedures weren't actually medically relevant at all, and it was actually within my right to refuse those examinations. (Astorino, "Brought to You By"; also see Astorino, "Intersex 'Treatment'")

Astorino's account of enduring humiliation and pain at the hands of fatherlike doctors for no health reason clearly draws attention to the fact that the curative violent practice of dilation is fuelled by phallogocentrism as well as compulsory dyadism and heterosexuality. In addition to doctors dilating children to make them "fuckable" (Triea 143), parents may also be instructed by doctors to dilate their children. As Emi Koyama explains, in this case "usually the mother is required to 'dilate' the vagina with hard instruments" (2).

Instituted Sexual Abuse

Many forms of curative violence intersex people are subjected to, including dilation, are instituted sexual assault and abuse. As Koyama posits: "Adult intersex people's stories often resemble that of those who survived childhood sexual abuse: trust violation, lack of honest communication, punishment for asking questions or telling the truth, etc. In some cases, [such as dilation] intersex people's experiences are exactly like those of child sexual abuse survivors" (2). Dilating children is not simply like sexual abuse; dilation unequivocally constitutes "institutionalized sexual abuse" (Driver qtd. in Arana 31; also see Guillot, Bauer, and Truffer; Orr, *Exorcizing Intersex*, "Sexual Assault").[2] These children are touched, examined, and penetrated against their will by their doctors and mothers, who are compelled to perform this abusive act as part of their gendered caregiving responsibilities and sexist understandings of how abuse occurs.

These systemic and systematic sexual abuses are, however, not readily recognized as abuses and are, therefore, difficult to deinstitutionalize and convict (Orr, *Exorcizing Intersex*). Dilation is not immediately understood as sexual assault or abuse because it is a medical prescription. Even though dilating a child for a prospective penis is absurdly heterosexist and misogynist, it folds into the powerful story of medical cure and is, thus, obscured. As Orr explains elsewhere: "The context ... renders the assault invisible and prevents so many from recognizing it *as* sexual violence .... the medical context in which these abuses occur and the assumed expertise we associate with doctors function as institutional protection to those who commit [doctors and mothers] (or prescribe [doctors]) the act of assault" ("Sexual Assault").

We acknowledge that medical professionals and mothers performing dilation do not think they are sexually abusing children, even though many intersex people testify to the contrary. The crux of this failure to recognize "is that those who have the power to determine what counts as abuse also have the power to ignore the claims of sexual abuse" (Orr, "Sexual Assault"). Medical professionals have the authority to determine if medical prescriptions constitute sexual abuse. It is also relevant that mothers, rather than fathers, are instructed to dilate their children, which obscures the sexual nature of this form of assault. Fathers, and men in general—not mothers or women—are typically (and understandably) assumed to be the perpetrators of sexual violence. While mothers and women can commit acts of sexual violence, men are more likely to be perpetrators of sexual assault and abuse. Hence, calling mothers to dilate their children disguises assault as maternal and medical care.

Conclusion

The mutilation and abuse of intersex people by their mothers at the advice of endocrinologists and other specialists echo the familiar social expectation of mothers to pursue the direction of medical experts for their own good and the good of their families. Challenging the many cultural assumptions and expectations that lead well-intentioned mothers to dilate their intersex children has the potential to stop the abuse. The culture of silence, abuse, shame, and unquestioned medical authority surrounding intersex is changing because of the invaluable work performed by intersex rights movement activists and scholars (Costello; Cameron; Viloria; Davis; Pagonis; Koyama; Cornwall; Astorino; Chase; Briffa; Holmes; Kessler; Karkazis; Magubane; Bastien Charlebois; Accord Alliance; Intersex Initiative; OII Intersex Network; AIS-DSD Support Group; Intersex Human Rights Australia; Stop Intersex Genital Mutilations; InterACT). Nevertheless, there is evidently more pragmatic and theoretical work to do to successfully undermine medical professionals' godlike authority and expert status. Eliciting the experiences of mothers themselves on the issue may further complicate the extent to which mothers resist or follow professional advice and how they interpret the consequences of compulsory dyadism for themselves and their children. These investigations will not only involve recognizing the sexually abusive nature of curative violence and intersex medical management but also acknowledging and grappling with the fact that mothers continue to be part of this management process and that their experiences are not well known. Accepting these facts is difficult; the medical institution, doctors, and mothers are symbols of healing, protection, cure, and care. We can challenge the promulgation of mind-body disabilities by bearing witness to intersex people's testimonies, by recognizing that intersex folks are the authorities on their experiences of curative violence, by no longer institutionalizing unethical and unsubstantial notions of medical cures, and by doing the necessary restorative labour intersex people require.

The work of the intersex rights movement to destabilize medical authority over people with intersex variations is significant beyond the experiences of intersex people. Mothers are incited to pursue established medical practices for their children who are coded as having a disorder or being disabled. Testimonies of intersex people help us understand how mothers of children deemed pathological and in need of cure are put in impossible positions with respect to their social roles as advocates, nurturers, and healthcare providers. Regrettably, when mothers become the instruments of their children's pain and (sexual) abuse, they significantly erode the mother-child relationship. It is particularly sad that pathologization and curative violence occur so early in the life of an intersex infant, risking the child-mother relationship from its tender start.

Theories of maternal responsibility and care would gain nuance from intersex people's testimonies. This testimony underscores how a care relationship always harbours violent potential (Kelly; Watson, *Accumulating Cares*). Though sometimes difficult for care theorists to acknowledge in their work on mothers who are already in precarious positions, care can empower and oppress. Only if the care relationship is questioned for its potential violence towards pathologized mind-bodies and people who are vulnerable to their caregivers can the voices of people with disabilities, or people who inherit mind-body disabilities from institutional medicine, be centred. An explicitly antiableist and anti-interphobic theory of care and maternal responsibility is required to challenge the medical industrial complex and status quo arrangements of power and abuse. Challenging the social disciplining of mothers and their disproportionate care labour responsibilities is not antithetical to challenging carer authority and power over carees, as the testimonies of intersex people require we consider.

Endnotes

1. The term "body-mind" is employed in this paper to resist the Western, Cartesian tradition of conceptualizing the mind and the body as distinct entities. To quote Eli Clare, the expression "body-mind" recognizes "both the inextricable relationships between our bodies and our minds and the ways in which the ideology of cure

operates as if the two are distinct—the mind superior to the body, the mind defining personhood, the mind separating humans from nonhumans" (xvi).

2. Highlighting the fact that intersex people and endosex women who have endured sexual abuse both report being touched and examined against their will, Karsten Schützmann and colleagues compared the mental health of intersex people and women who have experienced abuse. They report that both groups of people exhibit similar self-destructive behaviours and body-mind disabilities, such as depression and anxiety.

Works Cited

Accord Alliance. *Accord Alliance*, www.accordalliance.org/. Accessed 2 Feb. 2017.

AIS-DSD Support Group. *AIS-DSD Support Group*, www. aisdsd.org/. Accessed 24 Apr. 2017.

Arana, Marcus de María. City and County of San Francisco. *A Human Rights Investigation into the Medical 'Normalization' of Intersex People: A Report of a Public Hearing by the Human Rights Commission of the City and County of San Francisco.* San Francisco, 28 Apr. 2005.

Alexander, Tamara. "The Medical Management of Intersexed Children: An Analogue for Childhood Sexual Abuse." *Intersex Society of North America*, 1997, www.isna.org/articles/analog. Accessed 13 Apr. 2019.

Apple, Rima. *Perfect Motherhood: Science and Childrearing in America.* Rutgers University Press, 2006.

Apple, Rima. "Medicalization of Motherhood: Modernization and Resistance in an International Context." *Journal of the Motherhood Initiative*, Apr. 2014, jarm.journals.yorku.ca/index.php/jarm/article/view/39323/35652. Accessed 4 Apr. 2019.

Astorino, Claudia. "Brought to You by the Letter I: Why Intersex Politics Matters to LGBT Activism." *Autostraddle*, 23 Sept. 2013, www.autostraddle.com/brought-to-youby-the-letter-i-why-intersex-politics-matters-to-lgbt-activism-192760/. Accessed 1 Mar. 2017.

Astorino, Claudia. "Intersex 'Treatment' Trauma and Sexual Abuse Trauma: Not So Different." *FullFrontal Activism: Intersex and Awesome*, 18 Jul. 2010, fullfrontalactivism.blogspot.ca/2010/07/intersex-treatment-trauma-and-sexual.html. Accessed 1 Mar. 2017.

Baillargeon, Denyse. *Babies for the Nation: The Medicalization of Motherhood in Quebec, 1910-1970.* Wilfred Laurier University Press, 2009.

Bastien Charlebois, Janik. "Sanctioned Sex/ualities: The Medical Treatment of Intersex Bodies and Voices." *ILGA International World Congress*, 27-31 Oct. 2014, Mexico, pp. 1-30, old.ilga.org/documents/BastienCharlebois_2015_SanctionedSexualities_TheMedicalTreatmentOfIntersexBodiesAndVoices.pdf. Accessed 27 Sept. 2017.

Bauer, Markus, Daniela Truffer, and Karin Plattner. *NGO Report to the 2nd, 3rd and 4th Periodic Report of Switzerland on the Convention on the Rights of the Child (CRC). Intersex Genital Mutilations: Human Rights Violations of Children With Variations of Sex Anatomy.* Mar. 2014, intersex.shadowreport.org/public/2014-CRC-SwissNGO-Zwischengeschlecht-Intersex-IGM_v2.pdf. Accessed 1 Feb. 2017.

Briffa, Tony. "Tony Briffa Writes on 'Disorders of Sex Development.'" *Intersex Human Rights Australia,* 8 May 2014, ihra.org.au/26808/tony-briffa-on-dsd/. Accessed 29 Mar. 2019.

Cameron, David. "Caught Between: An Essay on Intersexuality." *Intersex in the Age of Ethics*, edited by Alice Domurat Dreger, University Publishing Group, 1999, pp. 91-96.

Cameron, David. "My Intersex Journey: From Awkward Teenager to Human Rights Activist." *21st Century Sexualities: Contemporary Issues in Health, Education, and Rights*, edited by Gilbert H. Herdt and Cymene Howe, Routledge, 2007, pp. 163-65.

Carpenter, Morgan. "Intersex health – Morgan Carpenter's presentation to Health in Difference Conference." *Intersex Human Rights Australia*, 22 Apr. 2013, https://ihra.org.au/22160/intersex-health-hid2013-plenary/. Accessed 28 Nov. 2019.

Chase, Cheryl. "Affronting Reason." *Looking Queer*, edited by Dawn Atkins, The Haworth Press, 1998, pp. 201-20.

Chase, Cheryl. "Hermaphrodites with Attitude: Mapping the Emergence of Intersex Political Activism." *The Transgender Studies Reader,* edited by Susan Stryker and Stephan Whittle, Routledge, 2006, pp. 300-314.

Clare, Eli. *Brilliant Imperfection: Grappling with Cure*. Duke University Press, 2017.

Clearway, Ajae, director. *One in 2000*. Polyvinyl Pictures, 14 Jun. 2007

Cornwall, Susannah. "Asking about What Is Better: Intersex, Disability, and Inaugurated Eschatology." *Journal of Religion, Disability, and Health*, vol. 17, 2013, pp. 369-92.

Costello, Cary Gabriel. "Interphobia—Not Cured by Hiding Us Away." *The Intersex Roadshow*, 12 Sept. 2010, intersexroadshow. blogspot.ca/2010/09/interphobia-not-cured-by-hiding-usaway. html. Accessed 17 Jul. 2015.

Davis, Georgiann. *Contesting Intersex: The Dubious Diagnosis*. New York University Press, 2015.

Davis, Georgiann. Interview with Casey Morell. "UNVL Professor Explores the 'Dubious Diagnosis' In Book About Intersex People." *KNPR*, 3 Mar. 2017, https://knpr.org/knpr/2017-03/unlvprofessor-explores-dubious-diagnosis-book-about-intersex-people. Accessed 3 Mar. 2017

Dreger, Alice Domurat, editor. *Intersex in the Age of Ethics*. University Publishing Group, 1999.

Greenberg, Julie A. "Health Care Issues Affecting People with an Intersex Condition or DSD: Sex or Disability Discrimination?" *Loyola of Los Angeles Law Review*, vol. 45, 2012, pp. 849- 908.

Greenberg, Julie A. *Intersexuality and the Law*. New York University Press, 2012.

Guillot, Vincent, Markus Bauer, and Daniela Truffer. *NGO Report to the 7th Periodic Report of France on the Convention against Torture. Intersex Genital Mutilations: Human Rights Violations Of Persons With Variations Of Sex Anatomy*, 28 Mar. 2016, intersex.shadowreport. org/public/2016-CAT-France-NGO-ZwischengeschlechtIntersex-IGM.pdf. Accessed 2 Mar. 2017.

Holmes, Morgan, editor. *Critical Intersex*. Ashgate Publishing Limited, 2009.

Inter, Laura. "Finding my Compass." *Narrative Inquiry in Bioethics*, vol. 5, no. 2, 2015, pp. 95-98.

InterACT Advocates for Intersex Youth. *InterACT Advocates for Intersex Youth*, interactadvocates.org/. Accessed 2 Feb. 2017.

"Intersex FAQ." *Intersex Initiative*, 29 Jun. 2008, www.intersex initiative.org/articles/intersex-faq.html. Accessed 29 Mar. 2019.

Intersex Human Rights Australia. *Intersex Human Rights Australia*, ihra. org.au/. Accessed 29 Mar. 2019.

Intersex Initiative. *Intersex Initiative*, www.intersexinitiative.org/. Accessed 2 Feb. 2017.

Karkazis, Katrina. *Fixing Sex: Intersex, Medical Authority, and Lived Experience*. Duke University Press, 2008.

Kelly, Christine. "Building Bridges with Accessible Care: Disability Studies, Feminist Care Scholarship, and Beyond." *Hypatia*, vol. 28, no. 4, 2013, pp. 784-800.

Kessler, Suzanne J. *Lessons from the Intersex*. Rutgers University Press, 1998.

Kim, Eunjung. *Curative Violence: Rehabilitating Disability, Gender, and Sexuality in Modern Korea*. Duke University Press, 2017.

Koyama, Emi. "Medical Abuse of Intersex Children and Child Sexual Abuse." *Introduction to Intersex Activism: A Guide for Allies*, compiled by Emi Koyama, Intersex Initiate Portland, 2003.

Lahood, Grant, director. *Intersexion*. Ponsonby Productions Limited, 2012.

Magubane, Zine. "Spectacles and Scholarship: Caster Semenya, Intersex Studies, and the Problem of Race in Feminist Theory." *Signs*, vol. 39, no. 3, 2014, pp. 761-85.

Magubane, Zine. "Which Bodies Matter? Feminism, Poststructuralism, Race, and the Curious Theoretical Odyssey of the 'Hottentot Venus.'" *Gender and Society*, vol. 15, no. 6, 2001, pp. 816-35.

Morland, Iain. "What Can Queer Theory Do for Intersex?" *GLQ*, vol. 15, no. 2, 2009, pp. 285-312.

"Not a Girl, Not a Boy—Intersex Documentary." *YouTube*, uploaded by Oh Jaume, 2 Apr. 2017, www.youtube.com/watch?v=R4mPGC-dNbQ. Accessed 14 Apr. 2017.

OII Intersex Network. *OII Intersex Network*, oiiinternational.com/. Accessed 29 Mar. 2019.

Orr, Celeste E. *Exorcising Intersex and Cripping Compulsory Dyadism.* 2018. University of Ottawa, PhD dissertation.

Orr, Celeste E. "Sexual Assault In Medical Contexts." *Impact Ethics*, 16 Feb. 2018, impactethics.ca/2018/02/16/sexual-assault-in-medical-contexts/. Accessed 29 Mar. 2019.

Pagonis, Pidgeon. "9 Damaging Lies Doctors Told Me When I Was Growing Up Intersex." *Everyday Feminism*, 3 Dec. 2015, everyday feminism.com/2015/12/lies-from-doctorsintersex/. Accessed 23 Nov. 2016.

Pagonis, Pidgeon. "The Son They Never Had." *Narrative Inquiry in Bioethics*, vol. 5, no. 2, 2015, pp. 103-06.

Preves, Sharon E. *Intersex and Identity: The Contested Self.* Rutgers University Press, 2003.

Schützmann, Karsten, et al. "Psychological Distress, Self-Harming Behavior, and Suicidal Tendencies in Adults with Disorders of Sex Development." *Archives of Sexual Behavior*, vol. 38, no. 1, 2009, pp. 16-33.

Stop Intersex Genital Mutilations. *Stop Intersex Genital Mutilations*, stop. genitalmutilation.org/. Accessed 29 Mar. 2019.

Tosh, Jemma. "The (In)Visibility of Childhood Sexual Abuse: Psychiatric Theorizing of Transgenderism and Intersexuality." *Intersectionalities: A Global Journal of Social Work Analysis, Research, Polity, and Practice*, vol. 2, 2013, pp. 71-87.

Triea, Kira. "Power, Orgasm, and the Psychohormonal Research Unit." *Intersex in the Age of Ethics*, edited by Alice Domurat Dreger, University Publishing Group, 1999, pp. 141-46.

Truffer, Daniela. "It's a Human Rights Issue." *Narrative Inquiry in Bioethics*, vol. 5, no. 2, 2015, pp. 111-14.

Villalobos, Ana. 2014. *Motherload: Making It All Better in Insecure Times.* University of California Press.

Viloria, Hida. *Born Both: An Intersex Life.* Hachette Books, 2017.

Wall, Sean Saifa M. "Standing at the Intersections: Navigating Life as a Black Intersex Man." *Narrative Inquiry in Bioethics*, vol. 5, no. 2, 2015, pp. 32-34.

Watson, Amanda D. "Quelling Anxiety as Intimate Work: Maternal Responsibility to Alleviate Good Feelings Emerging From Precarity." *Studies in Social Justice,* vol. 10, no. 2, 2016, pp. 261-83.

Watson, Amanda D. *Accumulating Cares: Women, Whiteness, and Responsible Reproduction in Neoliberal Times.* 2016. University of Ottawa Ph.D. dissertation.

Watson, Amanda D. *The Juggling Mother: Coming Undone in the Age of Anxiety.* UBC Press.

Wilson, Gina. "Intersex Genital Mutilation—IGM: The Fourteen Days of Intersex." *OII Intersex Network,* 25 Feb. 2012, oiiinternational. com/2574/intersex-genital-mutilation-igm-fourteen-daysintersex/. Accessed 19 Jan. 2017.

Chapter 7

An Intersection of Motherhood and Chronic Illness

Anna Johnson

In his exploration of the narratives of illness, Arthur W Frank writes of the potential "overdetermination" of chronic illness suffering. Whatever else you go through, the strain on your ability to cope is already overdetermined by the multiple factors in this background, or perhaps foreground, of difficulty, pain, effort, and all the rest. "All the rest" includes the frequent invisibility of chronic illness—the fact that it so often outstrips the allotted durations of sympathy and adjustments (only temporary measures, it seems) and becomes something unmentioned, unmentionable, socially inappropriate. Sometimes this invisibility is an act of survival, of getting on with it; sometimes it is a silencing when what is needed are words. Often it is both.

In this overdetermination of chronic illness, Frank suggests, chaos may be found, or rather entered, subsuming the subject's ability to narrativise their life, to tell themselves as a coherent story. So how are the difficulties of motherhood (and there are many difficulties) overlaid upon this already overdetermined situation of chronic illness? Below is one answer, one performative anecdote.[1] It is one of many (infinite, perhaps) possible answers but no less significant for that. As Donna Haraway suggests, "The only way to find a larger vision is to be somewhere in particular" (590). These anecdotal extracts are taken from a practice of creative life writing I began after the birth of my child. In this first anecdote both my child and myself are ill (I chronically, he in need of minor surgery), and in the anecdotes that follow, my child, my husband, and I are all ill and/or undergoing investigation for/living with neurodifference. These anecdotes may speak of small moments or realizations, but they suggest a complex intersectionality and the messy unevenness of life—particularly that of motherhood where bodies do not always feel fully differentiated and time can seem to fold back on itself.

The anaesthetist's eyes—as he directed me to the plastic chair set against the side of the hospital trolley—I'm not sure if it was compassion I saw there, perhaps just tiredness, something solemn. I am not good at lying, but in that moment, I feel the utter necessity of explaining out loud to my infant with full (and false) calm honesty that it is nap time, and he will have a little sleep now as I hold him, facing out, against my torso and they place the small mask over his face. His trust in me and his fascination in this new place and people mean there is no struggle, and perhaps he is too young to register the crack in my voice. I feel his body soften in my arms. I don't recall if I laid him down or they took him from my lap, but the next thing I remember I was broken down in the corridor, doubled over in breathless sobbing with the nurse standing by me, her hand on my back, waiting I suppose until I am consolable.

What if there is some danger in him? Something that will not be revealed until his precious skin is punctured. I could not bring myself to write in the few days before his minor surgery but now as he sleeps and breastfeeds and sleeps to recover, I can talk about this particular fear. I remember my ex's sister, as an adult, discovering an extra bone in her upper arm following an accident. And an anecdote recently shared by a friend about a head injury revealing an especially large occipital lobe, leading the injured to discover her visual perception of the world was, and had always been, markedly different from most. Then there's me. I have hypermobility syndrome, or, more accurately I think, I am hypermobile.

My tendons and ligaments, my veins, my responsiveness to pain killers and anaesthetics, my stomach (and more no doubt of which I am less chronically aware) are, to a degree, ineffectual.[2] But I look fine, tired now, but fine (after all, I have the velvet-textured "great skin" of the hypermobile and the slimness of a restricted diet) and went undiagnosed until the age of thirty-one, despite (or I sometimes feel because of) ten years of protestations that "something isn't right" and indications (mainly pain) since childhood. So I am acutely alive to the possibility of passing for well, physically as well as mentally, when in fact something is awry.

I feel ashamed writing about my condition. I don't know why. Perhaps the years of being patronised, disbelieved, and dismissed. Perhaps the self-preserving notion in many of "the well" that we choose to be sick (particularly the chronically so) and that I must, somehow, be doing this to myself, and enjoying it.

When finally (ten years after an accident from which I never recovered) my diagnosis was confirmed, I was invited to an information session about my condition. What soon became apparent at this gathering of chronically ill women (with the format of a corporate training afternoon) was that, for many, it was not the condition itself that was traumatic (although it can be hellish when un-managed) but the years of struggle to be believed that had altered us the most.

And then there is so much in motherhood that is hidden, so much waiting to be revealed, so many invisible processes that require so much faith. It is a faith that does not come easy (if at all) to me as someone who wants to see in order to know.

I felt as if he might simply deflate when cut.

Aside from the scattering of bruises on his shins (from fearless crawling) and the temporary, often theatrical, maquillage of food applied to his face at each meal, he has rarely been marked. Today, he is peppered with signs of yesterday's surgery, each of which pulls low at my stomach as I notice them again and again through my daily interactions with his body. In particular the tiny bruise and red-brown pin-prick to the back of each of his hands and the marker pen arrow, black fading to blue, on his left thigh. Also the unexplained bruise on his left cheek, two stitched incisions in his groin and grey, empty outlines from the heart monitors. But no secret was revealed. He is recovering well.

Frank suggests that "Medicine's hope of restitution crowds out any other stories." Not always. But in my experience, all too often. Of course, as I waited by the empty hospital bed for my son to be returned from surgery, I clung to that very restitution narrative—that medicine heals the sick, and we all move on (ideally unchanged). But that clinging took a tremendous effort and my grip was never secure because chronic illness is at odds with the restitution narrative; it is one of the "other stories."

I felt the absence of these "other stories" when I realized (years before my official diagnosis) that I had never been told I was chronically ill, although I had begun to be treated as such. I was still seeking a cure at the time—an answer that would allow me to enter into the restitution narrative and be fixed. Instead, I was offered a referral to a pain management class. No one ever said "we've given up, there's no cure, no treatment" to fix the (then unnamed) problem, and it took a long moment for the implications of the phrase "pain management" to sink in. So I am suspicious of what else isn't being said, and this changes my relationship to medical professionals and even to the architecture of medical spaces, which can inscribe relationships of openness or concealment and narratives of how our medical concerns are judged.

In the psychologist's office, as she evaded my questions about my son's behaviour, his (sometimes overwhelming) responses to others' emotions, I wondered about the curtain behind her. It covered, judging by its proportions, a wide but shallow window in an internal wall at roughly chest height—an observation window through which you might be watched playing with your child. The curtain reminded me of the decor of caravans, the kind we holidayed in in the 1980s, like the time we went to Scotland, and I was plagued with a recurring dream that my eyes fell out, or when we stopped for a night at a disused-race-track-turned-caravan-park, and my brother and I ran high up along the stalls, with the smell of concrete and metal and grass. The strange scale of the curtain, wide and short, and its oddness in the middle of an internal wall, not coming close to ceiling or floor, was exactly like something you'd find in a caravan, perhaps concealing a pullout table or a bed. Concealing something.

I managed not to cry at this visit, but then I didn't have to talk about my husband's health as he was present this time, and it was not mentioned. But still, the absence, again, of an answer to my direct question—in essence "should we be concerned?"—was maddening. As was the suggestion that I am perhaps too attentive to my child's needs (as of course the problem always lies in the mother). As was the feeling that the ugly ruched curtain concealed doctors. Presumably not at this moment, but that kind of intrusion, being watched, leaves its mark on the architecture that facilitates it.

It is perhaps not as obvious how my experience of chronic illness factors into this particular medical interaction, but it is there somewhere—in not being given a straight answer, in the idea that something clinical might in fact be entirely my fault, in being perceived as an "unreliable narrator" (Scarry), and in the uneasiness of an architecture for observation rather than communication. It seems to me that the uncertainties of motherhood—the working it out as you go along, the sense of never gaining a sure footing, especially when your infant is still finding language and you have barely slept in years—might be compounded by the limited sanctioned medical narratives and the, perhaps thoughtless or perhaps well-intentioned, restrictions of information this lack of narrative options entails. My own experience of being disbelieved for years and then being suddenly, and without ever being informed, deemed chronically ill, and finally, years later, being actually diagnosed makes me, as I said, acutely alive to possibilities outside the restitution narrative. And, moreover, acutely in need of the clear and open communication that observation windows, even unused and ineffectually hidden away by the most obvious of ruched curtains, seem to deny.

In her exploration of pain and its communication, *The Body in Pain*, Elaine Scarry describes pain as "more than any other phenomenon, [resisting] objectification in language." It seems to me that in sharing that resistance to "objectification in language" motherhood, my experience of its endless uncertainties, echoed my experience of being in pain and altered my understanding of both. Perhaps that resistance to language is exactly why I choose writing as a way of making sense of both motherhood and pain; in an attempt to pull these experiences out of their wordless isolation and to see these experiences spoken and, with any luck, heard.

There is a vulnerability, a risk, though, in attempting to voice these experiences that both evade language and have language stripped from them, withheld by their failure to fit sanctioned narratives. Sara Upstone writes the following in her essay "Against Health": "For many who are chronically ill, honesty and survival are brutal antagonists. The cruel art of self-deception is essential to push against the limits of a weakened, broken body. At the same time the loneliness of suffering pleads for recognition." To attempt to express these experiences might be to feel the full force of that brutal antagonism between honesty and survival; it might be to plead for recognition and be met with disbelief. The silence is structural, but I believe its resistance is worthwhile, essential even.

I would argue that honesty and survival are often "brutal antagonists" in experiences of motherhood, too, and can leave us backed into a corner with only the "loneliness of suffering." If not against "the limits of a weakened, broken body" (though for some, this is the case, especially at first), motherhood often entails a pushing against the limits of one's resources, physical or otherwise.

There was a certain necessary giving up I finally came to practice when he was eighteen months old. Life was too difficult, and suddenly I saw clearly that I needed to give up all but the essentials. I'm not sure I quite managed this, and after all, how do we decide what is essential? This writing could be the most or least necessary thing. In any case, I acknowledged the quiet state of emergency we were in, particularly with his father's health and what that really meant, and still means, for how, realistically, we might function. When I look back (as I am writing this a little out of time), I see this giving up as a descending calm that reminds me of walking home once through ancient streets covered in settled snow, quietened by its blanketing white yet made expansive by the simplicity of a single white surface. Our circle of travel narrowed: If you want to see us you have to come here. I know people don't understand, I fear I wouldn't have. But I have seen the limit of my energies, and what lies beyond, and I must stay within that limit. It is a hard limit, not a warning.

You may note I mention my partner's health again here. Partly, I don't go into detail about his health because that is not my story to tell, but also because this is the overdeterminacy of chronic illness. My partner's ill-health is just another thing on the list of things to be coped with. *And, and, and.*

In "Situated Knowledges," Haraway's seminal essay on the ideology of the voices with which we claim to speak, she argues for a "view from a body, always a complex, contradictory, structuring and structured body, versus the view from above, from nowhere, from simplicity" (589). Perhaps "Simplicity" is the place where only one symptom exists at a time, where only one partner is ill at a time, where mothers are not chronically ill. Clearly, I am not writing from Simplicity. What Haraway asserts is that *no one* is, even if their language and their ideology claim they are. Although some lives are simpler than others, few if any are simple, and there is no such place as Simplicity from which to speak. Haraway's vision of a way of situating ourselves that resists the limiting "ideologies of objectivity" (584) calls for "the joining of partial views and halting voices into a collective subject position that promises a vision of the means of ongoing finite embodiment, of living within limits and contradictions—of views from somewhere" (590).

My hope here is to offer one of these "partial views and halting voices" from a place of motherhood and chronic illness, sometimes from the edge of chaos.

Endnotes

1. I believe in Jane Gallop's description of the potential of anecdotal theory (theorizing with and through anecdote) as a form of "theorizing which honors the uncanny detail of lived experience" (2).

2. An early reader of this piece pointed out to me that my "responsiveness to painkillers and anaesthetics" cannot be ineffectual; simply, the drugs are ineffectual. Although I agree with her, I have not changed the text. What the text, as it is, reveals is the responsibility I felt to be well. The problem, as I saw it, wasn't the drugs (or the lack of understanding of how hypermobility, a primarily female condition, functions). It was me.

Works Cited

Frank, Arthur W. *The Wounded Storyteller: Body, Illness, and Ethics, Second Edition.* University of Chicago Press, 2013 (e-edition).

Gallop, Jane. *Anecdotal Theory.* Duke University Press, 2002.

Haraway, Donna. "Situated Knowledges: The Science Question in Feminism and the Privilege of Partial Perspective." *Feminist Studies*, vol. 14, no. 3, 1988, pp. 575-99

Scarry, Elaine. *The Body in Pain: The Making and Unmaking of the World.* Oxford University Press, 1987 (e-edition).

Upstone, Sara. "Against Health." *Versopolis.com*, 27 Nov. 2018, www.versopolis.com/times/essay/696/against-health. Accessed 30 May 2019.

Chapter 8

Mother Heal Thyself

Erin Northrup

I am nine years old. I am climbing a large oak tree in my babysitter's yard after school. It is a clear but windy day in May. I hear the familiar hum of my father's car coming down the road. I pick small pieces of bark off the tree and throw them in the grass below. After a couple minutes, I dismount the tree and see my father walking towards me. Although he has done this a hundred times before, today something is different; his steps are more purposeful, and there is something hidden behind his familiar smile. "Your mother has been accepted into medical school. We will be moving to Hamilton, Ontario," he says, his smile much bigger than usual. As children often do, I feign surprise and pretend to fall into a faint, landing in the soft grass. I lie there for a minute, feeling the prickly blades between my fingers. What does this mean? I picture our elderly, white-haired family doctor, Dr. Craig. His glasses are so thick they make his eyes look huge. He is kind and thinks he is funny when he looks in my ears and proclaims, "There are potatoes growing in there!" At the doctor's office, my mom is always serious; we're not allowed to spin around on the black-leather stool. She is always shushing us, and she listens carefully when the doctor speaks. I picture my mother with white hair, a white coat, and thick glasses telling other people's children that they have potatoes growing in their ears, and I laugh out loud.

Three months later, we are living in a new house in a big city. We used to live on a winding country road, but here the streets are straight, and there is a sidewalk that goes on forever. Our Grammie and Grampie take an airplane to visit us. We go for a walk and show them our neighbourhood. Even though my Grampie Jack is tall, he walks slowly.

I can hear him breathe, and I can hear the special clicking sound his heart makes. My mom says Grampie's heart clicks because it doesn't work properly; the doctors put a special device inside it called a Bjork-Shiley valve to help it work. My mom is so smart; she is learning all about hearts in medical school. As I walk beside my Grampie, I picture a little watch clicking inside his chest. I tell Grampie the sidewalk goes on forever. He smiles and tells me that my mom used to have a sidewalk in front of her house when she was a little girl. I like when Grampie tells me about my mom when she was little. I want to be just like my mom when I grow up. After Grammie and Grampie go home, my mom tells my dad that Grampie's heart is not good. She uses big words I don't understand, and she looks worried.

I am ten years old. I have just come inside from playing in the driveway with my sister. The phone rings, and my mom answers it. Her voice is serious; she starts speaking quickly, and she asks the person on the other side of the line a lot of questions. My mom calls my dad's name, and I hear her say the words "collapsed" and "CPR." It is one of my aunts who is on the other end of the phone. She has just told my mom that my Grampie has collapsed, and my Grammie is doing CPR. I run to my room and throw open my closet. People wear black to funerals, I think to myself. I grab a black dress with small red flowers on it. I am not sure if it still fits me, but I throw it into my duffle bag anyways. No one has confirmed it, but I know my Grampie is dead. I search through the closet for a dress for my younger sister, Julie. At ten years old, I am a serious and precocious child; this is my first experience with death, but I know it is final. My mom will need me to be a good girl and help her with my younger brother and sister; I find a dress for my sister and throw it into my bag.

My mom is crying now, and soon we are all in the car driving. We don't have the money to take an airplane. As we drive out of the city, my brother asks if my Grampie will be okay. My brother is only eight years old, and he doesn't understand the way that I do that Grampie is gone. I sit quietly in the backseat, watching the city lights fade away. I am filled with many questions. Why did the CPR not work? My Grammie is a nurse. She knows CPR. Why did the CPR not save my Grampie? I thought the doctor had fixed my Grampie when they gave him the clicking heart valve. Why did my Grampie's heart stop? I thought doctors saved people. I thought they fixed people. My mom is sad; she stares straight ahead with tears streaming down her face. I want to ask my mom why my Grampie is gone, but instead I look out the window at the endless stretch of dark highway. We drive all night, for seventeen hours straight, back to the place we used to live.

I am thirteen years old. My best friend, Tina, has been throwing up every day at school for months. Sometimes I go with her to the bathroom and wait outside because she is self-conscious that someone else will come in and hear her vomiting. Our teachers roll their eyes when she asks to go to the washroom multiple times a day. Tina has been to her family doctor; they tell her parents they think she has an eating disorder. Tina confides in me that she thinks everyone thinks she is crazy. Every day, she says she has a headache; I am worried for her. One day after school, I search through my mom's medical textbooks. I read the spines, searching for the appropriate text that will tell me what is wrong with my friend. For most thirteen-year-olds, the texts may as well be written in a foreign language, but their authoritative titles stand out like sign-posts in my head. I search each index for words like headache, bulimia, and vomiting. While searching, I come across a chapter on paediatric brain tumours. I show the book to my mom and ask her if she thinks Tina could have a brain tumour. My mom tells me I worry too much and sometimes teenage girls will make themselves vomit to lose weight. She asks if I think Tina might be trying to lose weight. I get angry with my mom, I thought she would be different because she is going to be a doctor, but instead she acts like every other adult. Tina is sick, and I don't understand why no one believes her.

Weeks later, I am getting ready to go skating with my friends. The phone rings, and it is my friend, Natalie. I can barely understand what she is saying between sobs. She tells me that Tina has gone blind and was rushed to the children's hospital where they discovered she has a brain tumour. She is in surgery to have something called burr holes so that hopefully she will be able to regain her sight. I hang up the phone and feel as though the wind has been knocked out of me. Wondering what transpired on the phone, my mom enters the room. "You were wrong!" I scream at her, "Tina has a brain tumour!" I search her face for reassurance that everything is going to be okay, and instead I am met with a look of quiet apprehension.

We soon learn that Tina has a medulloblastoma; her tumour is large, and she will need to have both radiation and chemotherapy treatments after her craniotomy. By chance, my school is mere blocks away from the children's hospital, and my mom is doing a clinical paediatrics rotation at the same hospital. Every morning before school, my mom and I visit Tina in the hospital. As the weeks and months pass, I become quite adept at navigating the children's hospital, but as the brightly painted corridors become more and more familiar, my friend becomes more and more a stranger. Tina gets progressively thinner and paler. Soon she is unrecognizable; her bald head and frail body remind me of the images of concentration camp victims from books and movies. One particular morning we enter the room to find Tina sobbing as her mother implores her to eat, trying to spoon thick pudding into her mouth. From the corner of the room, a nurse suggests it is time they consider a feeding tube. My mom and I quickly leave the room so as not to intrude upon the scene. Outside in the hall, I fall into step with my mom, and I ask her if Tina is dying. My mom is a resident now. I know she knows more about this situation than most mothers. If anyone can tell me the truth it should be her. I can see the pain on her face. She tries to reassure me: "Tina has some of the best doctors in the country..." but she trails off. She is trying to protect me. "I don't know," she says finally. Still, I feel she is withholding information. The air feels thick and anything but sterile.

I am seventeen years old. Two years ago, we left the city of Hamilton behind, and mom opened a bustling family practice in Sussex, a small farming community in rural New Brunswick, not far from where we used to live before mom went to medical school. I know my parents are relieved to have left the big city behind, but I, the ever-petulant teenager, am having a hard time adjusting to this recent move and to small town life in general. I feel stifled, and my new school is a lot more cliquish than my old one. I miss my old friends. I miss Tina, who is now in remission. Being a doctor's daughter in a small town feels like being Alice in *Alice through the Looking Glass*. I am an outsider. I cannot wait to leave.

Graduation is barely two months away when the house is startled awake by an early morning phone call. I roll over squinting at my alarm clock. It's 4:50 a.m. That's strange. Mom's not on call, I think to myself. There are muffled voices coming from the kitchen. I go down the stairs to find Mom hastily throwing her spare Littman stethoscope into a bag. "I can't drive you to school this morning; you'll have to take the bus," she says. "There's been some type of accident, a code orange; every doctor in town has to report to the hospital." I want to argue and tell her that I hate taking the bus, that none of my friends take the bus, and that it is embarrassing to sit alone. I want to ask her if she has remembered that she is on the Parent Committee for Prom and remind her there is a meeting tonight. Instead, I say nothing. My dad senses my irritability and looks at me disapprovingly. "Erin, you know this is serious," he says. The urgency of his tone tells me it is best not to argue on this particular morning.

At school, everyone is talking about the accident. A charter bus filled with children going to a music festival crashed outside town limits. There are whispers that some of the children died. I wonder if Mom can tell me what really happened. At lunch time, I walk to her office so I can talk to her. I remember I need to remind her about the Prom Parent Meeting anyways. When I arrive, the waiting room is fuller than usual. I hope she will have time to talk to me between patients. I wave to the receptionist and duck into Mom's private office. Mom walks in shortly, and I can tell she has been crying. I wait for her to talk. My mom is a person who has been granted an extraordinary understanding of human suffering. It is what makes her such a great doctor, but today the intensity of that gift is a heavy load to bear. Words usually come easily to Mom, but today her voice is thick and stilted. She explains how she arrived to pandemonium at the hospital. Frantic chaperones trying to account for everyone. Dead children. Colleagues trying to console worried parents thousands of kilometers away, over the phone. She wipes her eyes again quickly. She has to go she says. She has a busy clinic this afternoon, and patients from this morning are still waiting to be seen. I hug her goodbye. I leave quickly, knowing she won't be attending that prom parent meeting.

I am twenty-five. My husband and I are walking our dog on a sticky evening in early August. I am thirty-nine weeks pregnant with our first child, and I am hoping our nightly walks will bring on labour and put me out of this misery they call the third trimester of pregnancy. On this particular night, my plan works, and my water breaks. I call my parents, and they agree to meet us at the hospital. My husband and I arrive at the hospital shortly before midnight and are told that my membranes have indeed ruptured and we will proceed with a C-section, as scheduled. Although throughout my pregnancy I have disagreed with my obstetrician's insistence on a C-section, tonight I am resigned to the fact that this is how my baby will enter the world. I feel like I have waited my whole life for this moment—the moment I will become a mother. My husband is told to wait outside the operating room until I am given a spinal. The anaesthetist administers the spinal and drapes are placed. The obstetrician pinches one side of my abdomen, and I flinch. My spinal has failed to reach adequate anaesthesia; one side of my body is not frozen. I am rolled to the side, once, twice, three times. I am still not frozen. Doctors and nurses speak over me, never to me. The decision is made to move to general anaesthesia. I feel a sense of foreboding, as the mask is placed over my face.

I awaken in recovery, and my mom is there. I clutch my belly, panicked. Where is my baby? One of the nurses tells us my baby is fine, but he has been taken to the neonatal intensive care unit (NICU) as a precaution. I ask when I can see him. I am told that first I need to go the mother-baby postpartum unit. I can see my son in a couple hours. I am crying. If nothing is wrong, why can't I see my baby? Again, we are told my baby is fine; protocol dictates that I go from recovery straight to the postpartum unit. My mother is quiet, but I can see her growing disgust.

"I am a physician," she explains. "I am shocked at the utter disregard for the mother-infant bond. I do not understand why my daughter cannot at least *see* her baby." Thanks to my mom, on the way to the postpartum unit, I am taken through the open concept NICU. I am wheeled by slowly so that I can see my son sleeping in his isolette. I feel as though my heart will burst. I am a mother. I have a son and he is perfect. I can hardly wait to hold him. I am taken to the postpartum unit, where I try to rest for a couple hours.

My parents are in the hospital room with me. I am eating breakfast before I go to breastfeed my son for the first time. I cough and feel a popping sensation and a rush of blood soaks my incision dressing. Something is not right I tell my mom; she checks my dressing and quickly presses the call bell. She tries to be reassuring, but I am panicked. A nurse enters and takes one look at my dressing. A look of alarm crosses her face, and before we know what is happening, she is out the door grabbing the nearest obstetrician on the floor. A doctor I do not know begins probing my incision at the bedside. I've experienced a wound dehiscence she explains. I need to go back to the operating room now. I want to cry. I am tired. This was not how I pictured my first days of motherhood. I have not held my baby yet. I don't even know the colour of his eyes. I am supposed to go to the NICU and breastfeed my baby. Who will feed my baby? My bed is wheeled out of the room past my parents and husband. I realize I have not told my parents the baby's name; I was waiting until we could all be together with my new son. "His name is Jack," I say. My mom's eyes well with tears.

After my second trip to the operating room in the span of eight hours, we find out that the surgeon failed to cauterize an arteriole during my C-section, and the continued bleeding forced my incision open. When Jack is eight weeks old, my obstetrician calls me to apologize and inform me that the condition I was originally diagnosed with was a misdiagnosis; my C-section was performed in error. A comedy of errors, I think to myself. I look down at my nursing son and wonder how it is possible for a doctor's daughter to both abhor and revere medicine all at the same time.

I am twenty-eight years old. I am rocking my three-month-old son, Ben, while watching my husband try to wrangle our two-year-old son, Jack, out of his Halloween costume before bed. Halloween was three days ago. Sharks are cool, and pajamas apparently are highly overrated. I leave the room and call my parents' cell phone; I want to check in after remembering that Mom was having a CT of her sinuses today. If I don't call now, I know they will call me at the precise moment both kids are falling asleep and will wake them up. Do grandparents have a sixth sense for these things or is it karma? My dad answers, but his voice is muffled and almost unrecognizable. I ask about Mom's CT and he says, "We are still at the hospital; your mother is going to call you later." I say goodbye and hang up. Nothing my dad said was out of the ordinary, but I can't shake the feeling something is seriously wrong.

An hour passes. The phone rings, and it is my mom. Without pretense, she blurts out, "I have a large brain tumour." I suck in air so quickly; I don't know whether I am gasping or screaming or both. Mom had headaches and congestion; she thought she was having sinus issues; the threat of a brain tumour was never mentioned. Suddenly, the memory lapses, the headaches, and the clumsiness Mom had experienced over the last few months seem like blinking beacons pointing to her meningioma diagnosis. How was this missed? The conversation takes a clinical turn. Mom explains the tumour is large, over six centimetres. She has midline shift and parts of the tumour are calcified, suggesting it has been growing for a substantial amount of time. How can that be? Her neurosurgeons will attempt a complete resection, but it may not be possible because the tumour is invading the sagittal sinus. She informs me she will work in her clinic up until her craniotomy, which is scheduled for early December. "You can't possibly work," I tell her. That's not right. She protests and tells me there is no one else. There are patients and colleagues depending on her. There is already a shortage of family physicians in our small town, and her colleagues cannot take on her work in addition to their own busy practices. The irony is not lost on me: My mom is more concerned about the health of her patients than her own looming health crisis.

Mom's surgery date arrives; the pre-op area is eerily quiet. We are waiting for Mom to be taken to surgery. She holds Ben in her arms and asks me to take a picture. I look at it before showing it to her: my mother lying in a hospital bed, shorn hair, no makeup, grinning widely at her infant grandson. I wonder if this is the last picture of my mother I will ever take. I am unsure if I am more concerned that she won't be the same person after surgery or that she won't survive. Either way, I fear we will lose her. I hug her and walk out to join the rest of the family in the surgical waiting room. The hours pass, and finally the neurosurgeon comes in to tell us that surgery went well. They were able to remove most of the tumour but left a small section near the sagittal sinus. We should be able to see her soon.

Even after my experiences with my friend Tina's craniotomy, the temporary loss of speech and swelling, I am not prepared for Mom's appearance when I enter her intensive care room. Her head is misshapen, her face painfully swollen. She is agitated. Her speech is garbled and thick. The family is reassured that this is probably temporary, and it is. Mom is back to her normal self in a couple days, and we are incredibly relieved when she appears to have zero deficits after the surgery. Soon, she is checking her patient's lab results from her hospital bed. Mom is discharged from the hospital, and I host Christmas dinner a week later. There, Mom starts complaining of incisional pain, and because of its location, she cannot easily examine it herself. She asks me to look at the incision and take a picture of it for her. The incision is puffy and angry red with purulent drainage. She clearly has an infection. After a failed course of outpatient IV antibiotics, Mom is readmitted to the hospital for another surgery, this time to remove an infected bone flap. Further surgery is performed at a later date to insert a bone prosthesis. The rest of Mom's recovery is seemingly uneventful, yet we notice she seems to have some short-term memory deficits and some personality changes. I encourage her to take more time to heal before returning to a busy medical practice. Soon, however, colleagues begin to call, encouraging Mom to return to work. Some of them have taken on her patients. They do not say it to outright, but Mom knows they are overburdened with their own heavy workload; they need her practice to reopen in order to gain some reprieve. Despite my reservations, Mom returns to work, doing what she does best: caring for others instead of herself.

I am thirty-three years old. My husband and I have just recently moved back to Sussex, the town we were so eager to leave after high school. We missed the quiet familiarity of small-town life and want to raise our four children close to their grandparents. We move into the house across the street from my parents. It is a warm evening in September; the phone rings, and it is my father. "Can you come over; your mother is having a seizure. I have already called an ambulance." I keep my dad on the line and start running. As I leave, I can hear my eight-year-old ask if something is wrong with Grammie. Talk of seizures have become commonplace in our house. I struggle with the desire to be honest with my children but also protect them. I imagine this is the same way my own mother felt when raising me. I know now she didn't always have the answers. No one does. I walk through the door, and my mom is on the floor in the recovery position. She is breathing but unresponsive. Her skin is very grey. Dad tells me her seizure has lasted for over ten minutes now.

For the last five years, Mom's seizures have been woven into the fabric of our everyday lives. They happen during birthday parties, on Mother's Day, Thanksgiving, Halloween, Christmas, and then during busy clinic days in front of patients. Blood pressure cuffs are fumbled. Words are garbled. Roles are reversed, and patients call the emergency room for Mom when she has seizures in the examination room during their appointments. She starts medication, but still the seizures come and never with enough warning. I watch as her memory deteriorates. She approaches her doctors who are also colleagues, asking for advice. Is it safe to practice? Should she have neurocognitive testing before returning to work? She is met with blank stares, quizzical looks, and pats on the shoulder. "You're fine," they say. "We need you; your patients need you.

There is no one to take over your practice." I watch in frustration, as again the medical profession fails to rescue one of its own.

I am thirty-five years old. I am sitting on the porch with my mom. My two-year-old daughter, Audrey, toddles around at our feet. My mom's practice has been closed for a year. Her seizures had become too frequent and unresponsive to medication; her postictal states had become too debilitating, her neurocognitive testing too illuminating. She has reached the end of a career—one that she had sacrificed so much for and one she never had anticipated ending so suddenly. I worry about her. What is next for her? I also worry about myself. What is next for me? My maternity leave is over; it is time for me to go back to school and finish my graduate degree. My mom grabs Audrey and tickles her. Between my daughter's giggles, she asks me about my research topic. I explain that my thesis will explore the experience of mothers who have been failed by the medical system. It is my turn; I ask her what she has been doing with all her free time. She tells me she is writing a book, a memoir; part of it explores the lack of self-compassion that has become entrenched within the medical profession. She turns to me and says, "I always thought you would follow in my footsteps, Erin, even if you never became a doctor."

"I am, Mom."

"I know," she says.

Chapter 9

To Be or Not to Be a Woman in Medicine

Ajantha Jayabarathan

"If you were celebrating your two-year-old's birthday and got called into hospital, what would you do?" I was asked at my interview for medical school. "I would leave the party because it could be a matter of life and death for the patient," I replied. I was nineteen and wholeheartedly believed that a career in medicine would demand just that—the willingness to make personal sacrifices when it came to one's family. I felt the question was justified because entrance into medical school was fiercely competitive. If money and resources were being invested to train a female candidate, they needed reassurance that motherhood would not interfere with a woman's commitment to the practice of medicine. In contrast, male candidates could dedicate themselves more fully to medicine.

The profession in the eighties was predominantly male. They were supported by competent wives, who functioned much like single parents as they raised children and tended to their households. Bonding and caring for children were considered women's work. When I trained, would be fathers remained outside maternity wards while their children were born. Babies were separated from their mothers at birth and placed in rows of bassinets, where nurses kept watch over them. Women were deemed not ready to care for their own newborns. No wonder there was little tolerance for accommodating women and their biology within the profession. But I wanted to dedicate my life to a career in medicine and accepted that the price of admission was to prove that I would not come up short when compared to my male colleagues. I frequently reminded myself of this during the arduous years of training and practice.

Little did I know that my generation of female doctors would be responsible for what has been called the feminization of medicine. At first, women entered family medicine and paediatrics in increasing numbers because these fields offered flexibility to raise children. Female practitioners could share their practice with a female colleague and together manage career commitments as they birthed and raised their families. Gradually, women entered all fields of medicine. Outwardly, I was proud to be one of these women, but inwardly, it still gnawed at me that our biological underpinnings would disrupt our medical careers. The dissonance in my thoughts came from a fierce and misguided loyalty to the traditional practice of medicine and lack of experience in parenthood.

I brought this up to a male colleague. His wife was also a doctor, and they had four children. They assumed equal responsibility for raising their family and did not distinguish between male and female, generalist or specialist. He said:

> If it were not for women in medicine, I would be working eighty to a hundred hours each week and would not have time for our children or my family. I am grateful that your biology is showing men a different approach to their medical careers. Look at the incidence of suicide and substance use in male physicians. Consider their children, many of whom struggle to fill voids created by the lack of attachment to their parents. Why are we shortchanging ourselves and our families? Do they not deserve at least as much as we offer our patients?

Unfortunately, I had neither the maturity nor the experience to understand the wisdom of his counsel. Much like the journey of priesthood, I assumed the traditional male mantle of making the necessary sacrifices to have a successful career in medicine.

There was little time for anything but work during my training and early in my career. Working one in three on the call schedule meant that I had two days a week when I was not on call or recovering from being on call at hospitals. It was strenuous work and time passed quickly; but it was also gratifying. I slowly began to reap rewards—innovating medical practice, diagnosing, and managing complex patients, presenting at conferences, seeing my work published in peer-reviewed journals, training future doctors, and gaining skills to run and oversee medical clinics. At the age of thirty, I eventually found time to get married, and two years later, we prepared for the birth of our first child. It was thrilling to begin the next chapter that life had opened for me. I was accustomed to expertly juggling many balls and could foresee no problem with adding one more to the mix.

But in my third trimester, I was suddenly struck down by a knifelike pain in the lower abdomen and could not walk. I was worried about all the things that I knew could cause this. As I was wheeled into hospital, an experienced nurse watched me carefully and declared that my symphysis was separating. This joint holds together the two halves of the pelvis in front while the two sacroiliac joints hold it together in the back. She was so certain, that even before the obstetrician had seen me, she set out to help me. With quiet efficiency, she arranged for a sacral belt to hold my pelvis together and physiotherapy appointments to help strengthen my muscles.

The nurse's diagnosis was put to the test, when the obstetrician assessed me. "Nonsense, you just have a full bladder. Your pain will be gone once you empty it." I emptied my bladder and the pain disappeared! He made her cancel all the arrangements she had made. But I had a nagging feeling that she was right and that the pain got better because the bones shifted back into place, while I lay on the hospital bed for two hours. Who was I to believe? The nurse and my instincts or the obstetrician? I was well indoctrinated in the hierarchy within medicine, that specialists are experts and seldom questioned, even by other physicians. Having neither the confidence nor the language to challenge my colleague's diagnosis, I went along with his recommendation.

The day before his birth, my son's head measured at the upper end of the normal range on the ultrasound. "Do you think she can deliver him vaginally?" my husband asked. "Sure she can; nature has a way of making it happen," the obstetrician said reassuringly. But when my son's head was vaginally delivered, it tore the tissue apart, causing me to hemorrhage and go into shock. I was given a high spinal anesthetic for pain relief, which rendered me bedridden, barely able to hold my infant. Surprisingly, the obstetrician did not visit me in hospital, and no one explained what had actually happened to me. I was discharged home after a week, significantly weakened from blood loss. It was difficult to nurse and care for my infant, but I stuck to it with my characteristic determination. I learned firsthand that women entering motherhood endure suffering as a rite of passage and place the well being of their babies before their own.

I struggled to adapt to my new life in my weakened state. One morning, as I rolled over in bed, I felt a clunk and was paralyzed by intense, searing pain in the pubic area that took my breath away. But my baby needed to be nursed and I was alone at home. The only solution was to roll back and endure the pain as the bones shifted back into place. I then consulted with a physiotherapist who confirmed that my pelvis had separated during the delivery, and the two halves were hypermobile. She suggested a sacral belt to hold me together. So, the nurse had been right after all. My husband and I also realized that the obstetrician's reassurance about nature finding a way for women to deliver their babies did not hold true for us. He had not considered that our child was interracially conceived. My husband is Caucasian, from Northern Europe, and I am East Indian. My body was genetically shaped to carry and deliver an East Indian baby and was too small for my son's proportions. In my medical practice, I had not come across anyone with pelvic separation in pregnancy and did not recognize it in my own case. I then consulted with a second gynecologist, who clearly explained the extent of the damage and confirmed my assessment. I was greatly comforted by his kindness and candor.

I continued to have significant pain and was unable to crouch, squat, walk briskly or run without separation of the pelvic bones. Traditional practitioners could not help me, and my search led me to osteopathy and eventual recovery. That was the silver lining within this dark experience. I then incorporated osteopathy into my practice, and it helped hundreds of patients.

I returned to work when my son was four months old. I took a breast pump to work and added it to my juggling act. He was the light of our lives, and everything that was difficult paled in comparison with the joy he brought us. But his birth changed me, from the inside out. My experience with the specialist, who made two grave errors of judgment, and the resulting consequences to me and my family were undeniable. The lack of proper follow-up care was also evident. I acknowledged that the hierarchy in medicine can contribute to harm. The experience shifted my perspective, and I grew more confident in my critical appraisal of medical care.

When I prepared to have my second child, I made sure the care team was well informed. They were diligent and conscientious, and the delivery went without a hitch. I was thrilled to be home three days later, effortlessly nursing my baby with energy to spare. But on the fourth day, I developed a fever, chills, and significant fatigue. I needed my husband's assistance to get to my appointment with the obstetrician. "You know that you can feel very tired when you are nursing your infant night and day, don't you?" she said. "That is all this is. Don't worry. Everything is fine." I had enough confidence to ask, "Could this be due to retained placenta? " No," she said in a firm and dismissive tone. She offered no further explanation as she waved us away. But we insisted, and she grudgingly organized an ultrasound to satisfy us. My husband was furious, "Why is she treating you like this? You are a doctor, but she did not take you seriously and refused to believe you are ill. She is not even going to do the ultrasound urgently. How has she helped you?" It took a couple of weeks before the imaging was done, and I was much worse by then. The ultrasound showed a large piece of calcified placenta that needed to be surgically removed. As I sat waiting for the procedure, my obstetrician approached me. I believed she was coming to wish me well and felt comforted by the thought. Instead, I was shocked when she said, "They are not going to find anything but blood clots in there."

Before going under anaesthetic, I asked the operating gynecologist to tell me exactly what he found as soon as I recovered. "There was a large piece of calcified, undelivered placenta left behind," he said. "It appears we have let you down a second time." By then, there was infection in my blood, and I was admitted for intravenous antibiotics, which made my milk unsuitable for my newborn baby. As I lay in my hospital bed, the horror of the obstetrician's actions seared through me. How brazen of her to approach me before surgery to say they would not find anything of consequence? That there was nothing wrong with me. She had clearly missed the diagnosis. How could she justify her words? Was it a desperate move to avoid being sued? Why did it supersede acknowledging the harm done to me and my baby? It did not matter to her that I was a doctor and a colleague; I had to be wrong for her to be right.

My idols fell from their pedestals; their feet of clay finally revealed. Twice I had kept the time-honoured belief that the expert was always right and was proven wrong, with devastating consequences. They were fallible and some had learned to insulate themselves with arrogance and to disrespect the people they served. For the first time, I permitted myself to feel my anger and anguish. I acknowledged my deep disappointment in the colleagues that I had previously held in high esteem.

I had the revelation that each doctor's humanity is tested in their career. The grind of daily work can create blind spots and desensitize us. This process of getting callused can lead to dehumanizing those we serve and ourselves. I now recognize these as stages leading to burnout. But the two obstetricians also showcase gaps in medical training.

It is central to the practice of medicine to remain objective as we manage patients, and their needs. Over time, the walls intended to protect our objectivity, harden, and lead to loss of compassion, empathy, and humility. The gruelling training and on-call schedules lead us to disconnect from our human reaction and responses to patients. We can also disconnect from ourselves and become less responsive to our needs. We are not taught to debrief and reconnect with our core values and develop self awareness during our training. The lack of such mitigating strategies often results in damage to medical practitioners. We are trained to put out fires wearing protection that is barely skin deep.

We are also subject to unrelenting pressure to be accurate and timely in diagnosing patients and not missing anything that may present atypically. We must be up to date in our analysis and treatment interventions. We fear causing harm to patients; of being held liable if we miss something; but we are not shown how to manage the aftermath when we fall short of expectations. It is seldom modelled, that it is unrealistic to consider yourself infallible; that each of us can potentially harm patients and must minimise harm when mistakes happen; that we remain vigilant and humble to learn from mistakes. That we must guard against losing courage to face this reality in our careers.

The next event that affected me profoundly was the death of my own mother. Her loss is recent, and my grief is still deeply felt. Despite dealing regularly with life and death, it has made personal, the certainty and finality of death. My heart aches, as anguish squeezes my chest. My mother's loss has left a void in my life. Flashes of childhood memories are accompanied by pangs of deep sorrow and longing to have her back. Her loss brings to the forefront what my children will face when I am gone. It has raised the uncomfortable query whether I have been as present as my mother was in my life. Have I shared enough for them to remember and grieve about?

In my career, I committed to giving the shirt off my back to those in need. My life's journey has remained true to this cause and is riddled with compromises borne by my children, spouse, and extended family. Putting the needs of others above that of my family has come at a cost. I have not been present during my children's key periods of growth and achievement; it has often not been possible to see them at play. I was seldom home early enough, and the heavy workload was never far. They grew accustomed to me working on my computer and managing patient needs late into the night, early into the day, and into weekends. They are now grown, and nothing can bring back lost time. They reassure me that my absence helped them learn to be self-reliant and they have therefore developed agency. When she was seven, our daughter relied on her father to figure out how to pin her hair into a bun for ballet class. By eight, she could do it herself. But I am aware of the sacrifices my absence has demanded from them. They truly had no choice in this matter. They loved me and respected my chosen career enough to suffer in silence. The loneliness they felt searching for a mother who belonged more to others than to them is no doubt buried deep within. My children were fortunate to have a father who saw no distinction between the work of a mother and father—to be present in any way that your children need. "Sometimes one of has to give 150 per cent," he is fond of saying. And he has never complained that he assumes the lion's share of the 150 per cent.

I have asked my children and family forgiveness for being absent, for not being present, and for missing so much of their lives when they were younger. I also missed out terribly and denied myself the pleasure of being with them. How will they remember me when I am gone? Will they cry out that yet again I am missing when they need me?

My idealized commitment to my profession appears misguided from this newfound perspective. Despite being trained to assist others through motherhood, I did not grasp what it was to be a mother, until I became one. My adept juggling act kept me distracted from what was important. Unlike my patients who will find a replacement when I can no longer practice medicine, I am not replaceable for my children.

But in many ways, my children, and their need for me as a parent, also saved me from myself. They rescued me from the unbalanced approach to life and career that was modelled after the male-dominated world of medicine that I entered in the 1980s. Back then, being a woman in medicine felt like a problem; womanhood was a state that had to be transcended to gain respect and be valued. Remarkably, my less than stellar journey through motherhood taught me otherwise and enriched my practice of medicine. It helped me recognise the profound difference between delivering babies and what it means to give birth and become a mother.

If my daughter chooses a career in medicine and is asked the same question during the interview, this may be her answer.

> For a doctor, it is just as important to care for their own family as it is to care for patients. As a woman in medicine, there are many skills and values I bring to the table, that may be different than my male colleagues. Whether male or female, we deserve time to rest and time to step away from the heavy burden of responsibility that is placed upon us in this career. I watched my mother work day and night as a doctor and I want my own medical career to be different. Does your program value our wellbeing regardless of our gender? Does it teach us to balance our needs and those of our families with that of our patients? I would like to know how the system will support me to make sure that my patients are looked after while I celebrate my two-year-old's birthday.

Starting with the birthing process, women have collectively ushered in a new era in medicine. Now, both parents are present at the birth, and either one can be guided to cut the umbilical cord. Skin to skin contact, enabling the infant to crawl to the breast and nurse contributes powerfully to bonding and has ended the sterile medical processes of the past. Parental leave up to a year is available to support fathers and mothers when they start families.

There is growing awareness that our wellbeing depends on healthy work-life balance; and that balance within oneself is essential to achieving balance externally. A career in medicine, with responsibility for life and death decisions, demands supports that will allow us, as humans, to continue to offer our best to our careers. We must work in partnership with colleagues, not place them on pedestals and shy away from questioning them. The internet, which has made the science of medicine available to all who are curious, has further levelled the playing field. As patients empowered with knowledge about their symptoms present more fully as partners, they can better represent their needs and comanage their care.

I am witnessing the shift in colleagues, as they choose to reconnect with themselves and their families and grow more aware of the risks of burnout. The recognition of their own mortality, as well as their vulnerability to vicarious trauma, are shaping a protective, proactive approach to their career paths. This has caused an imbalance in the supply of medical practitioners and the healthcare system is grappling with consequences of tectonic proportions. Instead of developing collaboration and shared care of patients, the reduction in healthcare capacity is being addressed by increasing scopes of practice in a manner that breeds competition amongst practitioners and puts patients at risk. In Nova Scotia, doctors face lack of fair compensation, inadequate work resources, erosion of professional autonomy, and have been targeted with harassment when they speak out. Humanizing our dilemmas and offering locum support during vacation, supported sick leave, and pensions are yet to be realized.

The wellbeing of doctors and healthcare providers are fundamental to a healthy system of care. Physicians experience the onslaught of managing life and death struggles of patients, compounded by the seeming indifference of healthcare administrators, who know little about day-to-day challenges and are torn between managing the needs of the workforce and the demands of the healthcare system. We are audited, face complaints and get sued by the very people we try to help. When we miss a crucial diagnosis, we suffer as do our patients. We are ravaged by the stress and strife of our work, which affects our health and can lead us to an early grave.

But I remain optimistic and hopeful. Just as women entering medicine fundamentally changed the landscape of medical practice, I believe we are living through a revolution of change in healthcare. Nova Scotia is being disrupted by calls for critical appraisal of the results from policies and regulations created by government, healthcare administrators, bureaucrats, and academics. We are collectively demanding better and going through the pains of birthing a new system of healthcare.

As for me, I work hard to maintain a better work-life balance. I am less likely to offer the shirt off my back to others, since it would put my own survival in jeopardy, and I would no longer be able to assist them. There are grave reminders all around, as patients and colleagues succumb to illness, infirmity, and death. I embrace the time I have with my family and do my best to fill it with memories that we can all cherish. I recognise that all we truly have is the present. Lessons learned as we remain present through trials and tribulations add to our resilience and ability to handle life's challenges.

As I reflect on my journey, nearly thirty-five years after it began, I realize that the lessons left for me to learn were outside any medical school lecture hall or hospital experience. I am profoundly grateful for what motherhood has taught me. It humanized me and shed light on all that makes life meaningful. It has guided me to advocate for change in the healthcare system, so that all of us can flourish—doctors, patients, mothers, fathers, children, and families.

Chapter 10

Mommy's Operations

Hannah Feiner

When the students in my Portfolio group at the University of Toronto imagined their lives after finishing medical school, they sounded so certain. Most were clear that they would be married and in their desired residency spot. The question of children was not a matter of if but when. We launched into the often-repeated debate about whether it was better for a female doctor to get pregnant as a resident or staff. I love tutoring Portfolio, a reflective practice course for medical students. Throughout my own training, I dreamed about what it would be like to be a doctor: powerful, benevolent, upper middle class. Ten years after graduation, I am fortunate to be a physician, a wife, and a mother. But I didn't anticipate that these roles would be turned on their heads. I am also a patient. I, too, have needed mothering.

Through medical training, I often had tension headaches. On the wards, I carried ibuprofen in my fanny pack with my iPhone and patient list. In 2012, a year after I finished my family medicine residency, I had a migraine. I was surprised that my family friend Victor Toran (an otolaryngologist) insisted on brain imaging, as I hadn't had any worrisome symptoms. A month later, just as I was moving in with my boyfriend, Diego, I had an MRI. It showed that I had an astrocytoma, a tennis ball–sized malignant brain tumour. It couldn't be cured, but hopefully it would only be something of a chronic illness. Later that week, I had a craniotomy: Neurosurgeons sawed open my skull and removed the bulk of the tumour. Pathology showed a grade II astrocytoma. The natural history of this tumour is to degenerate into a GBM (glioblastoma multiforme or "greatest brain malignancy" as I memorized for surgery exams).

I had only been in practice for a year when I was diagnosed with an astrocytoma. My roles as doctor and patient have almost always coexisted. This dual identity has strengthened my commitment to family medicine, in which the physician-patient relationship is critical. I empathize with patients waiting for specialist visits, pathology reports, and insurance company decisions. Along with Paul Kalanithi, the neurosurgeon author of *When Breath Becomes Air*, I have seen firsthand how physicians should go beyond treating a patient's illness and attend to his or her emotional needs (Marchalik and Jurecic 2859). During medical training, I saw doctors as experts and care directors. My malignancy has connected me—person to person—with the patient seated across my desk.

My illness certainly changed me, but I didn't leave behind the dreams of my former life. I married Diego in 2013. My tumour behaved, and my oncologist gave us the green light to get pregnant. In 2014, Julia was born. We were blessed with our sweet, intelligent girl a month before my due date. Even during the excitement of pregnancy, I never left behind my identity as a patient. I was aware that as soon as I gave birth, I would go back to regular oncologist visits. When Julia was a few weeks old, I had my first MRI in fifteen months. The process was familiar— peace and stillness in the buzzing, thumping magnetic machine, the surreal, almost depersonalizing feeling of changing out of my hospital gown, the bubbles of anxiety in my chest rising and joining together in the days I waited for the results, and barely breathing as I rode the Princess Margaret Hospital elevator to the eighteenth floor. Before my pregnancy with Julia, my oncologist would tell me that I'd had what Diego called a "clean scan" and the anxiety bubble would release as I rode the elevator back down.

My first scan as a new mother showed that the remaining tumour had not grown in over a year. Months passed; Julia tried solid foods and learned to crawl, yet my anxiety bubble was still intact. I saw a therapist, Margot Feferman, who suggested that I couldn't talk my way out of uncertainty. She recommended a mindfulness-based stress reduction course, and I embraced it. I am currently taking my fifth mindfulness course in as many years. It has been life changing. I can now breathe through headaches, nausea, and guilt, knowing these feelings will pass. I can hope to be cured and accept my limited prognosis. In *Everyday Blessings: The Inner Work of Mindful Parenting*, Jon and Myla Kabat-Zinn reflect on mortality: "Perhaps the best we can do is feel the fleetingness of life and of our present moments and live inside them as fully as possible, hugging our children and delighting in their life, and feel at the same time the certainty of death, of life arising and passing away" (343).

When Julia was four months old, I returned to my weekly shift at The Bay Centre for Birth Control—the sexual health clinic at Women's College Hospital—just as I had done after my 2012 craniotomy. As a physician, the caring I provide for patients is well defined and time limited. This gives me a sense of control, as opposed to the limitless ministering required by my children and my patient role. Although it was empowering to step away from my patient and mother role and back into my professional identity, I relate to Amber Kinser's idea that bringing up children informs relationships with family, friends, and patients (124). Being a mother makes me a stronger family doctor. I can answer practical questions about parenting, provide hands-on assistance for breastfeeding, and in the sexual health context truly understand the importance of contraception.

My second daughter, Alice, was born in December 2016. When she was one month old, I had a seizure due to tumour growth. Then I had another craniotomy, followed by radiation and chemotherapy. I struggled with how to explain this to Julia, who was almost three years old. Diego and I spoke with Julia Broeking, a child psychologist. She helped us find the words to start a dialogue with Julia. In a study of mothers with cancer, Verena Bekteshi and Karen Kayser suggest that "Mothers and daughters could maintain a close relationship despite the cancer-induced stresses when they are engaged in open communication" (2379). I originally conceived of *Mommy's Operations* as a children's book after having spoken with Dr. Broeking. I had begun writing with the hope of starting a memoir. Dr. Colin MacPherson, a psychiatrist preceptor I had in medical school, emphasized his psychoanalytic role in the acute care unit as helping each patient fit their mental health crisis into their life narrative. This idea is echoed in *When Breath Becomes Air*: "The physician's duty is ... to take into our arms a patient and a family whose lives have disintegrated and work until they can stand back up and face, and make sense of, their own existence" (Kalanithi 166). I was about to have over a year off work with Julia in nursery school and a full-time nanny to help with Alice. It was time for my cancer-in-a-young-doctor memoir.

It was hard to get started. With time off work, I had imagined a scenario in which I would effortlessly switch between treatments, family life, and writing time. But the cancer treatments sapped my energy. My recent child-birthing, steroid-bloated, and patchy-haired body was a constant fixture of the B2 level of Princess Margaret Hospital. After hectic years of running my practice, scheduling the day was my major job. I rotated from a friend's car to waiting room to futuristic radiation machine to waiting room to friend's car. Hoping to be a more present parent, I planned my radiation schedule around Julia's nursery school hours, but I was often so tired that our nanny took Alice in the double stroller to do the pickups. I had stopped breastfeeding right before my craniotomy. I scrubbed my hands in the evenings after taking my chemo pills so the toxins wouldn't spread to my girls. Alice spent nights in the bassinet beside Diego while I slept with Julia in her princess-sheeted double bed. Maybe this is why Julia's voice came to me instead of my own. As Fiona Green suggests, "[Feminist mothers] strived for relationships based on respect, responsibility, and accountability.... They also acknowledged the experiences and knowledge of their children and encouraged them to talk about their own understandings and experiences with them in respectful dialogue" (165). While writing the version of *Mommy's Operations* that you will find below, I retold myself the exchanges we'd had with Julia about my illness. The process helped me to integrate my mother role with my patient role. The story is told in conversations between Julia and various adults. It ended up being too long for a children's book and too short for a play. It rests somewhere in between as creative nonfiction.

Throughout the maternity leave that became a sick leave, I was grateful to work my weekly shift at the Bay Centre for Birth Control and continue tutoring my Portfolio group. My physician role has become an important part of my self-identity. Eventually, I returned to my family practice in July 2018. As I write this introduction in May of 2019, I am balancing a return to chemotherapy, my medical career, and my family.

Mommy's Operations

1.

Julia was a spring baby. She was born after a winter in Toronto that people called the Polar Vortex. It was still chilly the month she was born, so her parents brought her home from the hospital in a pink bear suit. "Julia, Mommy and Daddy are taking you home today. We love you so much little baby. We can't wait to show you our house."

"Let's go honey, the car is across the street."

2.

Julia's sister Alice was a winter baby. Julia's mom put the pink bear suit on Alice when they walked Julia to nursery school.

"Mama, can I show my friends our new baby?"

"Sure Julia! We'll come into your classroom when we drop you off."

"Thank you!"

"Are you cold, honey? Do you want your neck warmer?"

"No neck warmer! I am fine."

3.

After Julia got home from nursery school, her mom made one of their favourite snacks: apple smiles. Alice was too little to eat, but she was allowed to be with her sister during snack time.

"Julia, I want to talk to you. Do you remember when Mommy had an operation when Alice was born? They made a cut in my tummy to take out the baby."

"Yeah."

"Next week, I'm going to have another operation."

"Why Mommy?"

"There is something growing in my brain that the doctors want to take out."

"Something growing? What is it Mommy?"

"It's called a tumour."

"A tumour? Are you going to be at the hospital again?"

"Yes, my love. I'm going to stay in the hospital for a few days after my surgery."

"So the doctors and nurses can check on you?"

"That's right, Julia. Just like when I had Alice."

"Who will be with me?"

"Daddy, Grandma and Grandpa will be here. They'll take you to school every day and tuck you into bed at night."

"I want you to put me to bed, Mommy."

"I will, for sure when I get back from the hospital."

4.

On the day of her mom's operation, Julia's dad picked her up at nursery school, so he could drive her to the hospital. He took her to the gift store.

"Daddy, is my Mommy at this hospital?"

"Yes Julia."

"I want to see her now!"

"She's almost done her surgery. Why don't you choose a present for her?"

"Mommy will love this pink balloon. Can I buy it for her, Daddy?"

"That's a beautiful balloon, Julia. After we buy it, why don't we take the elevator up to Mommy's room?"

"I want to push the button."

5.

Julia and her dad took the elevator to the ninth floor. A nurse at a big desk told her dad which room belonged to her mom.

"Here we are Julia. They will bring Mommy here when her surgery's all done."

"When her surgery is done?"

"Very soon, honey."

"Daddy, who's that lady?"

"She's the other hospital patient who will share this room with Mommy."

"I'm scared Daddy! Pick me up!"

"Come Julia. Daddy will hold you tight, tight. tight."

"Scared! Scared! I want to go home!"

"Do you want to wait outside the room for Mommy?"

"No hospital! Go home! Go home!"

"I'll take you home, Julia."

6.

Julia's mom did not come home for the whole school week. On Saturday morning, Julia was playing with Alice when her dad's phone rang. It was her mommy.

"Julia, Mommy wants to talk to you."

"Hi."

"Hi Julia!"

"Mommy, are you coming home today?"

"I can't come home for a couple more days. How about Daddy takes you to visit me in the hospital today?"

"The hospital?"

"You can have Old McDonald's for lunch and bring it to my room to eat."

"I want a chicken meal."

"Of course, honey."

"Mommy, can Alice come to the hospital as well?"

"No sweetheart. Only big girls are allowed. Grandma will watch Alice."

"Okay Mama."

7.

Julia's dad drove her to the McDonald's across the street from the hospital. He ordered a chicken meal for Julia and a hamburger for himself. Julia carried her box all the way up to her mom's room.

"Hi Julia! I'm so happy you came to visit! Come give your mom a hug!"

"No. I want to stay with my daddy."

"That's okay, honey. Mommy loves you so much."

"Momma, why you in a hospital bed?"

"Everybody stays in a hospital bed. Remember, I stayed in one when I had baby Alice."

"I love your eye, Mommy! Why you painted it pink?"

"Thanks Julia! It's just pink because this is the side I had the operation on."

"I want a pink eye just like you, Mommy."

8.

On Sunday, Julia's dad said she could visit her mom after she got dressed. Julia chose her clothes carefully—a long sleeved shirt to keep her warm and her favourite pink leggings.

"Hi Mama! I came to the hospital to visit you!"

"Hi Julia! I'm so happy to see you!"

"I like your headband, Mommy. Why you wore a pink one?"

"Because pink is your favourite colour."

"Thank you, Mommy. I want to have a pink headband as well."

"Of course, Julia. Did you know I'm coming home tomorrow? I'm so excited to be with my girls!"

"Tomorrow? Are you wearing your hospital gown to get home?"

9.

Even though the next day was Monday, Julia did not have school because it was a holiday. Early in the morning, Julia heard Alice making noises in her crib. She called for Daddy to bring her baby onto her princess bed.

"Daddy, is Mommy coming home today?"

"Yes, she is, Julia."

"Alice, our mommy is coming home! She wants to be with her baby and her Julia."

"Mommy will be very happy to be with her girls."

"Daddy, who will check on me when you pick up Mommy?"

"Grandma and Grandpa will stay with you and Alice."

"Can Grandma help me change into my princess dress? Mommy will love it if I'm wearing a princess dress."

"Of course, Julia."

10.

Julia and Alice liked having their mommy back at home. Julia's grandma stayed in the guest room so she could help. Julia made sure her mommy woke up every morning so they could play together before school.

"Come Julia, time to get ready."

"Mommy, I want you to take me to school and pick me up."

"I will take you to school Julia, but Grandma will pick you up."

"Why Grandma will pick me up?"

"I have an appointment this afternoon, Julia."

"But I want you to pick me up!"

"I know, honey, you want Mommy to pick you up every day."

"Yeah. Why you have appointments, Mommy?"

"I go to appointments so I can get better and better every day to be the best Mommy that I can for you and Alice."

11.

After Julia turned three, it was spring. Her mom still went to a lot of appointments. She tried to go when Julia was in school so they could be together as much as possible.

"Good morning!"

"Mama! Your hair growed back!"

"Oh no sweetheart, this is pretend hair. It's called a wig."

"Why you need pretend hair?"

"My hair isn't going to grow back for a while, so sometimes Mommy wants to wear pretend hair. Do you like it?"

"I love it Mommy! It's so beautiful!"

"Thanks, Julia."

"Is it your last appointment, Mommy?"

"Not yet sweetheart."

"When will be your last appointment?"

"Not for months and months, honey. The doctors want to keep giving Mommy medicine for a long time."

12.

When Alice was six months old, she needed a checkup. One day after school, Julia got to help her mom take the baby to their paediatrician.

"Hi Julia! How are you?"

"My mommy has a headband because the doctors took her brain tumour. She had two operations. One for getting out baby Alice and one for her tumour. She has pretend hair we call a wig."

"Wow Julia, you've had a lot of things going on. You sound like a very brave girl."

"Yeah, but Alice isn't a brave big girl like me."

"She isn't?"

"Nope. She's a brave baby."

Works Cited

Bekteshi, Venera, and Karen Kayser. "When a Mother Has Cancer: Pathways to Relational Growth for Mothers and Daughters Coping with Cancer." Psycho-Oncology, vol. 22, no. 10, Oct. 2013, pp. 2379-85., doi:10.1002/pon.3299.

Broeking, Julia. Personal interview. January 2017.

Feferman, Margot. Personal interview. May 2015.

Green, Fiona Joy. "Feminist Motherline." *Feminist Mothering*, edited by Andrea O'Reilly, State University of New York Press, 2008, pp 161-76.

Kabat-Zinn, Myla, and Jon Kabat-Zinn. *Everyday Blessings: The Inner Work of Mindful Parenting.* Piatkus, 2014.

Kalanithi, Paul. *When Breath Becomes Air.* Random House, 2016.

Kinser, Amber. "Mothering as Relational Consciousness." *Feminist Mothering*, edited by Andrea O'Reilly, State University of New York Press, 2008, pp 123-40.

Marchalik, Daniel, and Ann Jurecic. "Breathing Lessons: Paul Kalanithi's *When Breath Becomes Air.*" *The Lancet*, vol. 388, no. 1062, 10 Dec. 2016, p. 2859.

MacPherson, Colin. Personal interview. July 2007.

Toran, Victor. Personal interview. July 2012.

Chapter 11

Inner Turmoil: The Interconnectedness of Mothering and Doctoring

Sally J. Bird

It is Friday evening at 6:00 p.m. I am standing in my driveway with a baby on my hip, a toddler screaming that she "WILL NOT GO!" and a sad-looking five-year-old. My husband was supposed to be home by now to take the five-year-old to basketball. But he is late. He just called to say that there is a patient who is in crisis and needs an admission. With great frustration (maybe rage?), I am hurriedly packing everyone up to take my son to the game. Even though this scenario regularly occurs in our family, I had concluded that my husband was going to be late... again... too late. Now I am rushed, cranky, and irate. It is an unpleasant scene. I am near tears—because in addition to the current miserable situation in the driveway , I cannot stop thinking "How did I get here?".

This was never the plan—to be the harried mom with a bunch of kids, angry with her partner for coming home late from work. It was supposed to be me who was late coming home from work after saving people's lives and doing compassionate and important work. How did I end up being the one waiting at home losing my cool?

Growing up, I had a recurring daydream. I would walk home from the bus stop, imagining my life as an adult. I would arrive home after a long day of work at the hospital. My house would be filled with warmth and light, and inside would be a wonderful man and a gaggle of happy children. Supper would be ready, the kids would be cute, and the house would probably be tidy (I didn't pay attention to those things as a teenager). The man would kiss me hello, and the kids would come running. The dream always contained the same three elements: I was a doctor, I was a mother, and I was married.

I did not recognize it then, but I was imagining my father's life. My mother, a physiotherapist, gave up her career when we moved to the small island where my father was going to be the sole paediatrician. He worked or was on call for work most of the time. My mother, an incredibly capable woman, kept it all going at home. They felt that the children should have someone at home to compensate for how often my dad was gone. Although my home example was of traditional gender roles, it never occurred to me that it was the way it had to be. It also never occurred to me that someone had to be at home making it all happen.

Every weekend, I went with my dad to the hospital to see his patients. I recognize now that it was to give my mom a break. I saw my future in this world: I couldn't imagine a more interesting career. It was meaningful, it was never boring, and it was rewarding. I have never wanted another career; I have always wanted to be a doctor. And a mother. Always.

I was elated, the day I received my acceptance to medical school. "My dream will come true!" was my first thought, followed closely by "I will always be financially independent and able to support my children." In the first moment when I knew I was going to be a doctor, my thoughts included my future children.

Choosing a specialty of medicine was an agonizing decision. Modern medical education has created a system in which students must choose their specialty path early, often before they have fully experienced all of the options. I had assumed that I would become a paediatrician and work in a rural location, like my father. Along the way, I discovered that I loved using my hands to perform technical procedures. Unexpectedly, I loved the operating room environment. I developed a passion for obstetrics and gynecology and set about applying to that program. However, I had a persistent worrying thought: Could I be both the type of mother that I want to be and the type of doctor? Thoughts of my own future babies still danced in my head. The obstetrical residents I knew were overworked, tired, and, as a result, appeared to be ill-tempered most of the time. A chance encounter with anesthesiology just before applications were due presented an unanticipated option. This specialty allowed me to work with my hands, be in the operating room, care for obstetrical patients and children, and remain slightly more in control of my life. I could imagine a life as an anesthesiologist and a mother. The anesthesia residents and most of the staff physicians I had met were happy with their work and not nearly as irritable as the obstetrical residents.

My boyfriend (future husband) and I applied to our preferred residency programs and began our residencies together in a large city. It was a harmonious cohabitation with both of us working long hours and studying. We made exactly the same amount of money. This is a helpful way to begin cohabitation—with financial and professional equality.

Residency was hard. It demanded more of me that I had ever known before. But it was also great fun. We were finally real doctors! I was working in the operating room and performing preoperative assessments, and as my experience increased, I gained more independence. I finally felt like a doctor. I loved it.

Residency, though, was where I first perceived a gender disparity in my chosen profession. Whether I had been in denial all the previous years of my life, or simply oblivious, I don't know. I am grateful that I was unaware until I was twenty-six because I can't predict how I may have been influenced as I worked towards my goals. Time and again, I witnessed female doctors, including myself, being treated differently by patients, nurses, and ward clerks. The women would regularly be forced to wait longer to gain someone's attention, have a surgeon interrupt their preoperative assessment, or have a patient say, "I'll just wait to decide that until the doctor arrives"—the assumption being that the female resident was not a doctor. My female coresident would complain about various frustrations to our male colleagues, only to have them look at us blankly. They were having a different experience. Residency also highlighted gender differences in my own relationship: how differently my husband and I would experience the road to becoming parents.

Having a baby in residency had never occurred to me and was not my plan. Despite my drive to be a mother, I didn't think a lot about when I would become one. Around the time that we got married, the beginning of our fourth year of residency, the media blitz on the increasing infertility of career women was blowing up. There were articles everywhere about how women were delaying having babies and then finding out at thirty-five or thirty-seven that perhaps they had waited too long. As I was turning thirty, this weighed heavily on my mind. What if I couldn't get pregnant later and missed my chance to be a mother? I had always taken the straight and narrow academic path, with my eyes firmly set on my goal of becoming a doctor. Was it time to deviate? Could I wait until I finished residency at thirty-one, followed by a year of fellowship and the time spent starting a new job, to have a baby? It suddenly seemed risky to wait. I was tormented by the knowledge that I wasn't ready to have a baby, but being a mother would trump being a doctor if I had to choose. Uncharacteristically for me, we took a chance on our honeymoon and came home pregnant.

I kept the pregnancy a secret as long as I could. I suspected that things would change; people would think differently of me if they knew. I had witnessed this happen to other residents. My pregnancy was revealed when I requested a change of assignment to avoid giving anaesthetics for patients undergoing radiotherapy. There is a risk of radiation exposure when looking after these patients—one that does not normally concern me, but it is something to be avoided when pregnant. My secret was out. I had to request to be excused for certain appointments, such as ultrasounds and prenatal appointments. People's attitudes towards me changed. Before I had been considered an excellent and hardworking resident, and then almost overnight, it was as if I were now considered lazy and not working hard enough—loafing off in the middle of the day. It was difficult. The equality of my husband and I was no longer, and I was resentful. Nothing had changed for him. Life went on as before. He wasn't missing work or being forced to ask for any accommodation, but he was still going to get to have a baby. This was the first inkling I had that things might be different for him, the father, and me, the mother.

Our son was born at the beginning of my fifth year of residency—nine months before the dreaded, all important Royal College exam. These exams are the culmination of all the years of study; without passing them, you cannot practice your specialty. It is as if the entire future of your life has come down to these few days of tests. The year of study leading up to these exams is perhaps the most stressful of a medical trainee's life (at least this is how it feels at the time), and now I was going to add a new baby on to this year. My mother-in-law was delighted, as we were making her a grandmother. My mother was terrified: Would her beloved daughter come so close to becoming a doctor, only then to do something stupid like staying home with a baby? My thoughts were focused on one thing: How could I get organized enough to manage it all?

Our son was a beautiful, healthy baby and we were enamoured. I was a mother and a doctor. But there was no elation. There were only thoughts of how to make this all work. I read books on sleep training. I breastfed but bottlefed breastmilk early to ensure that he would take a bottle while I studied. When the poor little guy was only four weeks old, I put my plans into action. I am the only mother in my circle who truly sleep trained their baby by letting the baby cry. I decided he needed a rigid, predictable sleep schedule. (Or, rather, I needed this to predict when I could study.) Fortunately, he was an easy-going baby who thrived on routine. I allowed him to cry it out, and he accepted his fate willingly and never really put me to the test with prolonged crying. The will power required on my part to do this was ever present for this baby. The exams loomed large, and I was convinced that if I did not do this, I would fail, and all my dreams would disappear. I could not be convinced otherwise.

My son's entire infancy was overshadowed and influenced by my need to work and to study. I went back to work when he was six months old. I could have taken a full year, but I was determined to sit the exams with my cohort of residents. We had become good friends, and I wanted and felt I needed their support to make it through the exams. I chose to leave my baby with a full-time nanny in order to return to my fifty-to-sixty hour a week clinical commitment and continue to study for the exams in the evenings. I wanted to write the exams on schedule, despite having a baby.

We were working and studying, and the baby was thriving. My dream had come true: I had a perfect healthy baby. Truthfully, I was missing out on his babyhood—not because I was away at work but because when I was home, I was thinking only of studying. One night I was sitting with him in his rocking chair, his soft warmth snuggled against my body, and I was thinking "Come on baby. Get sleepy. I have to study." And it hit me: What are you doing? This is a precious moment. You are lucky to have it, and you are wishing it away! I tried my best to be present with him at least at bedtime. It was hard. My eyes were still on the prize of becoming a doctor, and I had one huge hurdle left to jump.

Prior to our residency baby, we had plans of going overseas for a fellowship. Pregnancy and maternity leave meant a delay in finishing my clinical training, and although we had passed the exams, we now had a baby to consider. In the end, we furthered our training in the same city. This meant stability for all of us but mostly for our son. We kept his nanny and his life the same and continued our training. It was an acceptable alternative, but we missed our chance to spend a year living in another country, something I still reflect on today.

With the extra training I pursued, I became a paediatric anaesthesiologist. This subspecialty of anaesthesia combines all of my loves: anesthesiology, caring for children, spending time with families, and working in an environment where everyone puts the patient first. The world of paediatric medicine is kinder and gentler; everyone understands the need to take a bit more time for a child to be ready or for a parent to have that one last hug before their child disappears into the operating room.

After becoming a mother, I found myself regularly unable to dissociate my own role as a mother from the child in front of me. I viewed every parent and child duo as if it were me and my child. In some ways this was an improvement. I became more empathetic with my patients and families, and I developed more patience for them. I am also more emotional. I like to think that this makes me a better doctor, but I am not sure emotion is always beneficial in medicine.

In turn, these experiences have made me a better mother. As my years of experience increase, they force me to maintain some perspective. I am reminded on a daily basis that "there but for the grace of the universe, go I." Who knows what could happen? Today, I am the mother of three healthy children, but a car accident, a playground incident, or a sudden ominous diagnosis could change all that. When kids are being kids and I am being a cranky mom, I try to remember that I am lucky to have this chaotic house, to spend my Saturdays as a taxi driver, and to spend countless hours preparing food. I am not naturally prone to gratitude, my experiences at work remind me to be humble and thankful.

I believe work-life balance as an anesthesiologist is easier to achieve than in some other medical specialties. It is not without its challenges, and sometimes my definitions of "good mother" and "good doctor" clash. Both require presence—both physical presence and mindful presence. At times, they are incompatible with one another, and this I find excruciating.

When my youngest son was three, he was very attached to me in the way that many little ones are. (I once saw a poster in my hospital with the caption "Mother's Body = Baby's Natural Habitat." This perfectly sums up how he felt. Cuddles with me would bring him great comfort.) One evening he was sick with a flu; he had a stuffy nose, a high fever, as well as aches and pains. He was miserable and sad. All he wanted was to snuggle on my chest in the rocking chair. The next day, I was scheduled to give an anaesthetic for a complicated and long (more than sixteen hours) neurosurgery case. I was worried about the case and my role in it. I had to be rested and prepared for the next day. I popped in the ear plugs, left my husband to deal with our sick wee one, and went to sleep. He woke up many times that night, crying out for mommy. I heard it but pushed my ear plugs in farther and went back to sleep. That night I chose another child's needs over my own child's. Although I have never questioned whether it was the right decision, it was painful and felt terribly wrong.

Now I am ten years into my professional career. We have three children and established careers. I am "living the dream" as my mom enjoys reminding me. My dream didn't include the bad-tempered mom in the driveway, yelling at her kids to get in the car while cursing her husband under her breath. In my fantasy, I had overlooked the fact that in order for home to be a peaceful place, someone has to keep the home. I did not marry that person, nor did my husband. Thus, we struggle to find the right balance of work commitments and home commitments. We struggle constantly with the push and pull of who will say "yes" to professional opportunities and who will say "no" in favour of home commitments. More often than not, I say "no" to work and "yes" to home. I am always weighing the effect my work commitments will have at home. As the children get older, this will likely (hopefully?) shift, but for now, I do my best to excel at my profession while regularly prioritizing home.

As it turns out, my intuition that life an as anaesthesiologist would better support my overall life goals was correct. One of the benefits of my specialty is that there is a group of us who share the same specialized skillset. Although I may want to be at work for a certain patient or case, I know they are in excellent hands with my colleagues. This is unusual freedom in medicine. It means that I can work part-time and not feel like I am letting my patients down. It means I can take a day off to chaperone a class trip or to hang out on a PD day. I believe that this is sowing the seeds for a long-lasting close relationship with my children.

And I hope that the professional opportunities will still remain when I am able to engage more fully.

I am envious of my husband going to work and not thinking about home, not receiving texts about kids' arrangements, and not reading emails about upcoming recitals. When he is at work, he is present at work. When he is home, he is an excellent partner. However, I am downright jealous of his confidence that the children will be fine and that making another professional commitment won't detract from home commitments or family relationships. Secretly, I wonder if he feels that way because he knows I will always prioritize home over work. I will never know because I am unable to pull back from home more than I already have. My definition of a "good mother" centres around presence. I want to know all the gritty details of what's going on in school and choir and basketball, which sometimes requires engaging in what is happening at home when I am at work and definitely means reading all those damn emails. My husband said we play to our strengths, and one of mine is managing details, both in my work and at home (his is special projects both at work and at home). I know he is right. Sometimes I wish he wasn't.

My roles as mother and doctor are indelibly intertwined. One is always influencing the other. Decisions about how to engage at work are always influenced by home and vice versa. I am more compassionate with my patients but sometimes less compassionate with my children. They have to be very ill for me to take them seriously. At the same time, I am constantly aware that life is fragile, and everything can change in an instant. I feel like I live odd paradoxes all the time. I will stay late at work for a case when it appears that handing over the care of the patient could affect the outcome, but I will firmly set a limit and leave early on a day when I committed to a school event. I am callous about my children's flus and colds and scrapes, but I am acutely aware that their healthy status can change in an instant.

My life as a mother working in medicine is not what I dreamed it would be when I was young. Unbeknownst to me, that dream was likely unattainable to anyone but a man of a previous generation or a woman with a partner who wants to stay home or have a career secondary to their spouse. And it is definitely not attainable for someone of my personality, who hovers on the line of control freak. I am always envious that my husband doesn't read emails in a timely manner and that his phone doesn't ping at work with kid-related messages. My mind would be freer and life at work would be more peaceful. I could say "yes" without weighing consequences when an opportunity arises. It wasn't meant to be that way for me. I wanted to do both—be a mother and a doctor. This requires compromises in both roles. For me, the compromise is this: The roles remain intertwined in both their influence and also within my time. I engage with home while working and with work while at home. It is messy and frustrating and beautiful and fulfilling.

Chapter 12

Narratives of Mothers' Medical Experiences on the Internet: A Challenge to Medical Dominance?

Darryn Wellstead

Contemporary ideologies of intensive mothering and total mothering, which draw heavily on a neoliberal narrative of personal responsibility, position mothers as accountable for "anticipating and eradicating every imaginable risk to their children" (Wolf 72; Hays; MacKendrick; Reich; Villalobos). Although such ideologies suggest mothers rely on experts, such as doctors, for information, access to experts is limited. It is, therefore, unsurprising that many mothers turn to the internet, which is readily available, for health advice and social support (Zaslow). The internet now rivals physicians as a primary source for health information, and women make up a large proportion of users (Larsson; Lemire; Rainie; Statistics Canada). Researchers have illustrated that people use websites, listservs, and online support groups for health information and social support, but beyond that, many gaps in research remain (Audrain-Pontevia and Menvielle; Hardey; Kivits). They know little about how people use social media to talk about health, and even less is known about the broader impacts of a health praxis that is increasingly internet driven.

Some researchers have suggested that the internet may open up new opportunities, pathways, and networks that challenge medical dominance, yet our understanding about how this works is limited. Michael Hardey found that patients use information on websites to advocate for their health needs in medical interactions, whereas Emile Zaslow shows that women's use of an email listserv opened up space for a "revalorization" of feminine ways of knowing and thinking, positing that such activities may pose a challenge to medical dominance. Similarly, in their study exploring the use of online health communities, Anne-Francoise Audrain-Pontevia and Loick Menvielle argue that the more empowered patients become, the less committed they are to their physician. Although these are important findings, their utility is limited. Such general studies, with broad conclusions, do not tell us anything specific about which parts of medicine are being rejected and why.

An interesting development tied to the expansion of health information on the internet is the rise in complementary and alternative medicine (CAM) use, particularly among women (Canizares et al.). The global expansion of the antivaccination movement has also been linked to the internet and has gained traction through social media in particular (Smith and Graham). Such phenomena give us reason to consider how participation in online spaces might not only empower individuals but also pose a challenge to medicine more generally, both in terms of its dominance as well as its authority.

To complicate matters, studies of health-related issues (like vaccination) on social media have tended to focus on Twitter and public Facebook pages, where conversations are polarized and are often inflammatory, even though most people likely do not look to such public spaces to discuss personal health matters. Whereas public platforms are sometimes described as akin to the wild west, Facebook groups have been described as a sort of sanctuary from "clickbait, recipe videos, and salesy spam" (Holmes), offering users more intimacy, collegiality, and productive dialogue. This may help to explain why Facebook group membership increased 40 per cent in 2018 (Holmes). To my knowledge, no research has examined health discussions in Facebook groups or has explored them as potential sites for a renegotiation of medical knowledge and authority.

Acknowledging that mothers are often the key health decision makers in the family (Bird and Reiker), my study explores how mothers use divergent Facebook groups to talk about health and medicine. I find that such groups are indeed important sites through which mothers both challenge and uphold medical dominance and that online interactions in these spaces do in fact shape offline medical decision making. In this chapter, I show how medical authority is frequently questioned in ways that are not universal across groups but rather are context specific. I suggest that although grievances aired in these spaces do reflect problematic areas of medicine, they are also influenced by group focus.

The goals of this chapter are threefold: (1) to explore the nature of discussions around medicine in online communities; (2) to explore the ways in which such discourses either challenge or uphold medical dominance; and (3) to theorize about the potential implications of the role of medicine and mothers' health decision making more broadly.

About the Research

This chapter draws from an eighteen-month study investigating how mothers use Facebook groups in talking about and making decisions about health. The study centred around two Facebook groups with contrasting ideologies—one focused on natural living ("the natural group") and the other focused on science-based parenting ("the science group").[1] The groups each had over six thousand members, and I was a member of both prior to beginning the study. The project was approved by the University of Ottawa Research Ethics Board (REB).

The research involved three distinct phases: (1) daily participant observation in the groups over a year-long period; (2) a critical discourse analysis (Wodak and Meyer) of conversations in the groups over a five-month period (examining a total of three hundred separate discussions); and (3) in-depth interviews with twenty-one mothers belonging to these and other, similar groups. In total, I interviewed eleven members of the natural mothering groups and ten members of the science mothering groups, for a total of twenty-one respondents. Over the course of my research, I accumulated nearly three thousand typed pages of data as well as many handwritten notes. I obtained consent from interview participants as well as for the use of unique and detailed quotations from the discussion groups.

About the Groups

The purpose of the natural group is to help people who are interested in living more naturally, which was defined by participants as eating organically, choosing natural household products, reducing waste, growing or foraging for food, and making nature a part of one's lifestyle. Although the group is open to anyone, the majority of members are white, English-speaking mothers from Canada and the United States (US). Most of the posts tend to relate to health matters, with a smaller proportion dealing with parenting concerns and other lifestyle-type questions, such as gardening, foraging, and reducing waste. Health-specific posts cover a wide range of topics, including questions about natural remedies, diet, boosting one's immune system or other medical concerns; advice for locating a healthcare provider or dealing with doctors; and the occasional question about more obscure matters, such as genetic testing and protection from electric and magnetic field radiation. Ideologically, discussions in the group tend to appeal to nature, with the overwhelming message being that what is natural is better in terms of food, health interventions, medicines, and practices. So although the group does not take a formal position on vaccinations, conversations on the topic tend towards an antivaccination stance.

The science group identifies itself in its description as an "evidence-based" parenting group; it views parenting as something that ought to be informed by scientific and/or peer-reviewed research. The majority of members are mothers, but the group administrators state explicitly in the group rules and announcements that they are inclusive of fathers, transgender, and nonbinary parents. Although the group is more racially diverse than the natural mothers, they are still predominantly white. Questions from the group tend to be evenly split between parenting (e.g., children's book recommendations or dealing with tantrums) and health (e.g., information on fluoride, dealing with allergies, or experiences with genetic testing), although specific medical advice is strictly prohibited. Ideologically, the group gives primacy to scientific knowledge and also tends to favour the advice of medical authorities, such as the Centers for Disease Control (CDC) and the American Academy of Pediatrics (AAP). They take a strong provaccination stance, regularly critiquing those who hold antivaccine perspectives.

Findings

Among the conversations of medicine in these online spaces, several themes emerged that address my question of how medical authority is upheld or challenged. In this section, I review my findings around these discussions. I argue that even though medicine maintains a stronghold in maternal discussions about health, its dominance is challenged in distinct ways according to each group's focus. In the natural group, medical authority was challenged through frequent posts highlighting distrust and dissatisfaction with medical providers. However, members regularly upheld the value of medicine for acute or urgent issues. In the science group, medicine received regular and vocal support and was viewed as a major authority on health-related matters. However, mothers still challenged medical dominance around major grievances related to sexism as well as specific concerns, such as infant feeding, childbirth, fatphobia, and bodily autonomy. In the following section, I present these themes through highlighting a selection of information-rich discussions, which illustrate the variety of ways in which medical dominance is either challenged or upheld.

Natural Group: Distrust and Dissatisfaction

Discussions about health and medicine in the natural group frequently took the form of what I broadly categorize as distrust and dissatisfaction narratives. These generally appeared as shorter anecdotes in which a member describes an interaction with a physician or medical provider that left them unsatisfied. They were often posted to solicit advice in navigating a medical condition or health-related issue. Within this category, several themes emerged, including dismissive care providers, pushy care providers, and limits to physician knowledge.

Dismissive physician narratives were frequent and varied widely, but they generally reflected the view that patient concerns were brushed off or not taken seriously. One member asked the group for advice about digestive issues: "I would rather not go to my family doctor, as he is quite useless and rather rude to me, dismissing everything I say." Here, the authority of the physician is called into question, as the mother simply decides that his advice can be discarded on the basis that he is useless and rude.

Similarly, members frequently shared stories about pushy physicians (or other healthcare providers). These stories tended to be shorter and less detailed and were sometimes couched in other conversations, particularly those relating to vaccinations, like this post from Amelia, a young mother of an infant:

> I'm looking for a naturopath in the area for my daughter, husband, and myself, but mostly for my daughter. Specifically, I want someone who doesn't just hand out medicine but instead does the proper testing. I would love if they are anti-vax, as I'm tired of doctors forcing their vaccination opinions on me. I would prefer someone who respects choice.

Amelia's quote illustrates elements of the ideology of individualist parenting (Reich), a consumerist approach to healthcare (Lupton), and the rejection of standard medical practice in favour of alternative practitioners. Doctors are framed as "pushy" and as "forcing" their "opinions." Medical dominance is rejected, as Amelia looks to the group for recommendations on a naturopath who would abide by her personal standards of proper procedure and choice.

A final theme among negative experience stories was the common sentiment that there were limits to physician knowledge. This was a frequent trope in conversations around vaccination as well as nutrition. For example, it was common to see comments that expressed that "doctors aren't trained in nutrition." Such statements directly challenge medical knowledge and authority, with the implicit presumption that others—even mothers themselves who have spent enough time doing research—can be better informed about nutrition than doctors. As one mother noted, "Part of living naturally is not always listening to medical professionals blindly and seeking better opinions." Here, the mother takes up a blind-faith metaphor to challenge the authority of medical professionals, suggesting that there are better options if one wants to live naturally. In discussions of vaccination, members sometimes claimed the following: "Doctors are not trained in the dangers of vaccines at all. All they know is the vaccine schedule, and that is it. Please do more research." The authority and knowledge of doctors are questioned, and doctors are framed as limited in their ability to understand and administer vaccines. In such cases, mothers are encouraged to be skeptical of physician advice and to rely instead on themselves to "do their own research." The knowledge they gain through conducting research is implicitly more trustworthy than the knowledge of physicians.

When mothers left a medical encounter dissatisfied with their experience, they often were encouraged by others to trust their gut and to push for what they wanted. Jen, a mother of three young children, posted in the group to ask for advice on how to go about requesting an MRI. Although multiple doctors had diagnosed Jen with anxiety, she remained convinced that she had an underlying medical issue that was being ignored. Another member, Alissa, replied:

> I'm so sorry you're going through this! I bet you the reason WHY you have anxiety is because they aren't taking you seriously! I had a similar thing happen with my daughter where doctors just didn't listen to us. We ended up going to the hospital eight times this month in order to get them to believe us. I hate that we have to be so persistent and relentless, but that fight is 100 per cent worth it. You will know in your gut when things aren't right. Trust it! It won't steer you in the wrong direction. Move forward and demand answers. Trust your intuition and let that guide you.

This is an example of what Zaslow refers to as a subtle challenge to medicine and a revalorization of feminine ways of knowing. Jen's feelings are validated, and she receives encouragement to continue to fight to have her health concerns recognized in way that will satisfy her. The multiple doctors' diagnoses are not authoritative knowledge but hurdles to be navigated. The implicit suggestion is that the only person Jen can count on in this process is herself. Jen alone must trust her intuition and advocate to have her concerns taken seriously. When medical authorities do not validate one's concerns, the recommendation is to continue to push until heard. In other cases, mothers were encouraged to do their own research and/or consult alternative practitioners, such as naturopaths.

This finding was further reinforced through the individual interviews, during which several mothers noted that "medicine has its place" but also valorized alternative medicine and treatments as a viable and even preferable option. In response to the question: "Generally speaking, how do you feel about Western or 'conventional' medicine?", there were a variety of similar answers:

Mira: I feel like it has its place, and I feel like it's really good for when you have no other option or when you really really really need it. But I think it doesn't have to be the primary. I think the primary should be natural healing when at all possible because there are other side effects.

Laura: I feel like there's a place for Western medicine, and I think that also, you know, when my kid gets something, like say my kid got a staph infection, it's not like I'm just going to rub some organic fuckin' honey on it and be like, "It's gonna be totally fine," and we'll just shove you full of kombucha and give you some probiotics, and… No, like, there's a time and a place when like, you need medicine.

Erin: I think Western medicine has its place. I mean, my baby would not be with us today if it wasn't for Western medicine. She absolutely would've died. I absolutely would've died. Both of us would've. In a sense, that experience has humbled me a little bit more to Western medicine because I was, I wouldn't say anti-Western medicine, but not really so much of a fan of it.

Vanessa: I don't think Western medicine is all bad. I just feel more research needs to be done and proven and that doctors need to be honest with patients at all times. We shouldn't have to research ourselves.

Thus, despite the prevalence of distrust and dissatisfaction narratives, members also reaffirmed the place of mainstream medical doctors. For example, mothers with sick infants or serious medical issues were regularly advised by group members to see a doctor or go to an emergency room. Health ailments deemed to be of a more severe nature (such as issues with eyes) were often referred to mainstream practitioners. This finding suggests, as other scholars (Canizares et al.) have documented, that despite increasing interest in alternative and holistic approaches, the place of biomedicine remains firmly entrenched, even among more natural-minded mothers.

Science Group: Overall Approval but Major Grievances

Overall, and in contrast to the natural group, the science group was more consistently supportive and enthusiastic about medicine. Members would regularly make statements such as "my doctor/

pediatrician told me..." and would encourage each other to "talk to your doctor" for a wide range of issues, both major (e.g., possible postpartum depression) and minor (e.g., a diaper rash). Although individuals sometimes seemed frustrated that they could not request medical advice in the group, the majority of (vocal) members supported this position, suggesting that medical advice provided over the internet could be irresponsible or even dangerous.

When members sought out specific information, group members and administrators tended to privilege medical knowledge or information from health-related authorities. For example, in a discussion about fluoride in the science group, members pointed to the advice of their paediatrician, dentist, as well as the American Dental Association (ADA):

Karen: When do I need to start supplementing fluoride?

Sally: Our paediatrician prescribed fluoride drops at my son's six-month visit.

Meagan: I'm pretty sure my daughter started getting fluoride drops around three months.

Niki: Here's what the ADA says: [quote excluded]

Eliza: Once the first tooth comes through, you should schedule a dentist appointment. They can give you all the information you need to care for baby's teeth.

Karen: Thank you all! I love that I can ask a question about fluoride in this group and not hear horror stories.

Occasionally, medical authority and knowledge were called into question. Challenges to medical dominance tended to revolve around major grievances, such as sexism and fatphobia in medicine. When such critiques were levelled against medicine or individual doctors, members would discuss or refer to scholarly research to make critiques of how medicine was practiced. Samantha said the following:

Doctors are susceptible to the same biases as the country at large. While ruling out vaccines as dangerous is obviously stupid, all that stuff etc... on the flip side, there is solid research to show that you get worse care if you are fat because doctors over-ascribe your conditions to your weight. There are also plenty of case studies that indicate that doctors are less likely to believe women about their symptoms and thus put them at greater risk of health complications. There are legit reasons for people to be wary of doctors; it's just unfortunate that antivac folks have clouded that reality with their woo[2] bs.

Members also challenged medical authority when doctors gave advice that the group deemed to be inconsistent with scientific knowledge and/or peer-reviewed evidence. One mother described her experience taking her child to a walk-in clinic, where the doctor said the baby's respiratory syncytial virus was due to her "not breastfeeding." The members expressed anger at the physician's shaming of the mother and remarked that "what the doctor said is bullshit." Several members posted links to science-based sources of information to refute the doctor's claim. One mother, Nicole, linked to peer-reviewed research in her support of the poster: "There are a handful of studies regarding BF [breastfeeding] and bronchiolitis. They do not point a finger at non-BF as a cause of bronchiolitis but rather shortened hospital stays with bronchiolitis and allowing moms to BF during the hospital stay. My guess he's only reading headlines and not actually reading the scientific articles."

Here, the doctor's knowledge is questioned, and it is suggested that he may not have a complete understanding of the issue. Similarly, another member comforts the poster: "Don't let him make you feel guilty. Clearly, he doesn't understand passive immunity. I'm sorry your baby is sick!" In such cases, when doctors were perceived to have fallen short of expectations, particularly around evidence-based care, members would sometimes suggest that the mother find a new doctor. This was particularly the case if doctors espoused views that members perceived to be pseudoscience. For example, one mother posted in the group that her doctor told her that food dyes can cause hyperactivity in children. Two members responded: "Woo. Find a new doctor." Thus, it seems that medical knowledge holds authority for members as long as it does not violate evidence-based knowledge or standards of care. Members sometimes posted in the group to get advice on what questions to ask when meeting with a medical professional. Typically, these sorts of screenings were meant to ensure that a physician followed an evidence-based practice and to avoid taking on a doctor who is "deep in the woo." These discussions reflect the emergence of a consumerist power dynamic, in which mothers hold the authority to determine whether a doctor meets an evidence-based standard of care (Lupton).

An additional way in which medical dominance was challenged was through the sharing of negative medical experience narratives. In this case, medical dominance was not typically challenged directly, but the groups provided an alternative means for mothers to make sense of and even reinterpret their experiences. Negative experience narratives tended to surface most often around major grievances tied to sexism. Here, personal stories were presented as anecdotes to support broader claims. In such cases, grievances were not generally targeted towards individual healthcare workers but were attributed to specific ideologies and policies viewed as harmful for women. The most frequently mentioned grievances centred around the issues of infant feeding, childbirth, and bodily autonomy. These often occurred together, and members highlighted the cultural tendency to value women's bodies for what one member termed their "base biological functions." There was a strong sense of outrage over the moral imperative to breastfeed, and mothers tended to blame their individual maltreatment on broader ideologies and frameworks, such as the World Health Organization's position on breastfeeding and the US-based Baby-Friendly Hospital Initiative (BFHI), which promotes exclusive breastfeeding and rooming-in practices following childbirth.

Mothers' narratives around negative medical encounters elicited a sense of solidarity among members (evident through such comments as "I can relate" and "I had a similar experience") while also providing anecdotes to support broader claims being made. Such narratives described in great detail accounts of being treated poorly during and following birth and in conversations around breastfeeding and reproductive health. Such stories regularly addressed issues such as a lack of proper pain management, negligence in medical care, or an assault on bodily autonomy (which evoked particular feelings of rage among members). Rachael explained that she had a hospital lactation consultant hook her up to a breastpump without her consent while she was in the intensive care unit with a postpartum pulmonary embolism and stroke. She later filed a complaint against the hospital. Another mother, Christina, told a disturbing story in which she was repeatedly denied formula following her child's birth. She explained that eventually her husband smuggled it in but that the nurses "kept trying to take it after they knew." A nurse would come to the room every ninety minutes with a pump "to make me do it." She explains:

> Eventually, this became such a deep concern with my ability to take care of my child properly that they called child services, so a couple days after I got home guess who showed up on my doorstep? (We were in the hospital for almost two weeks.) Why? Because I said, "I can't." Obviously, [child services] and I had a chat over some snacks and drinks, I showed them that I was combo feeding and following closely. It was immediately declared unfounded. They did disclose that they had been following more and more of these cases recently.

> In hindsight, I could have been a better advocate for myself. I could have been firmer. I probably should have, but I was not at all well, and I was solo parenting a newborn while trying not to die myself. We continued to combo feed until she was one. First mostly breastmilk because if I hadn't kept on with that, there would have been more complaints—then (when I was less terrified that using formula would lead to her being taken away) mostly formula. I am an educated, privileged woman who is well versed in what advocacy is and what my rights are, but that goes out the window when you have five children and child services shows up because you have been reported as not caring enough because your breasts are not going along with the plan.

It is clear that Christina is engaged in a process of sense making around her traumatic experience. As she notes, she is "still not over it" four years later. She reflects on the pressure she received from healthcare workers and the traumatizing impact of having child services called on her because of her failure to breastfeed. She later notes: "I wish I had been in this group, or any similar—at that point. I was surrounded by helpful folks who wanted to send me lactation cookie recipes." Indeed, Christina's story is an example of how the sharing of stories in groups offers the opportunity for a sort of retelling of an experience from the standpoint of the patient, in light of broader discussions around sexism in medicine and ideologies that may be harmful. In doing so, mothers' experiences are no longer isolated but can be interpreted alongside the knowledge and experiences of others. This represents a subtle challenge to medical knowledge, as mothers are able assert the importance of their own experiences, knowledge, autonomy, and feelings in the face of a system which reduces mothers to their biological functions. As Christina notes:

> Still not over it, and she's going to be four soon. Shockingly, women bloody well matter. We are more than baby-making/baby feeding machines. I don't know why the current movement is to reduce us to those base biological functions, but no. We are patients, we are people, we are physical and have emotional limits. We are our own choices, our preferences, and our voices. Sometimes, we need some amplification of those voices—even those of us who are usually the outspoken, outraged, and empowered.

Interviews with mothers from the science group reaffirmed these findings. Mothers frequently noted that medicine was a good thing, but that there were problems relating to sexism, fatphobia, the profit motive, and access:

> Darryn Wellstead (DW): Generally speaking, how do you feel about Western or conventional medicine?

> Breanna: I have mixed feelings about it. I'm glad that it exists. I am glad that many of the tools that we have exist that have come out of it. I think that it is often discriminatory, and I think it's deeply problematic how profit driven it is in the US. But, like I said, I tend to try to treat it as a tool. So, like, if I'm going to the doctor's office, I usually—most of the time—try to go with a pretty good idea of what's going on with me and what I want to get out of it. Or what's going on with my child and what I'm hoping to get out of it. And there are some like individual practitioners I trust more, like I actually really like our paediatrician, but as a whole, I think the medical industry is an industry and is not particularly trustworthy or necessarily helpful. But I use it because… it's useful.

> Elizabeth: For the most part, I am for it, very supportive. There's been so many medical breakthroughs that have just been so helpful, for not just the US but for the world. And so I am

definitely, for the most part, supportive. There are definitely problematic aspects to it, such as... in the US, we don't have any kind of socialized medicine, it's a for-profit industry, and it can be very predatory. And a lot of people just don't get the care that they need because of the policies in place. My experiences as a uterus owner have been fairly negative, unfortunately. Female-presenting people often get subpar healthcare as opposed to male-presenting people. I've been dismissed for many of my problems just because they see me as a female.

DW: Can you give an example?

Elizabeth: An example would be when I went in because I was having pain during intercourse after having my daughter. Rather than trying to find a source of pain, I was told I should take some Advil a little bit before having sex, presumably for the rest of my life. The doctor I saw was a fatphobic misogynist. He told me he wouldn't help me with my incontinence because I was too heavy. And the fact that he did not care that I was in pain and just tried to make it so that I could continue having sex with my male partner that was in the room.

Discussion

Across both groups, discussions challenged the authority and/or dominance of medicine but not in universal ways. In the natural group, there is a sense of disenchantment with medicine, observed through narratives that emphasize distrust and dissatisfaction. Medical authority was frequently questioned and compared to other knowledge authorities, leading mothers towards alternative practitioners, such as naturopaths, and towards a reliance on their intuition and their own research. Yet medicine was regularly reaffirmed as "having its place," particularly in relation to more severe issues. Thus, although medical dominance is challenged and mothers are eager to pursue alternatives, mainstream medicine is still important to natural-minded mothers. In contrast, medical dominance is affirmed in the science group, where mothers look to doctors as a key source of authority on a wide range of matters relating to their own and their children's health. Occasionally, medical authority was challenged, when it was presented in ways members perceived as sexist, fatphobic, or otherwise harmful to mothers—for example, when bodily autonomy was denied or when women were reduced to their biological functions. The group vocalized their anger and spoke out against perceived maltreatment. In addition, some members challenged medical authority when doctors failed to give them scientific and/or peer-reviewed advice or treatment. Although the groups clearly reflect different overall views of medicine, the overall sense of frustration seems to resonate across both. Mothers are frustrated by medical encounters when they are dismissed, patronized, or feel that their needs (e.g., for care, pain relief, and bodily autonomy) go unmet. The importance of this last point should not be understated. These are valid concerns.

Future research should examine how such challenges to medical authority impact mothers' decision making for themselves and their families offline. Do members of the natural group more frequently reject doctor's advice after members tell them to do more research? Do members of the science group advocate for themselves more with an increased recognition that maltreatment may result from sexism? We might also begin to explore more specific questions around observable trends related to issues such as antivaccine attitudes. Are people who reject vaccines obtaining information from online communities, as some have speculated? If so, we should pay more attention to the persuasive power of challenges to medical dominance in such spaces. Understanding the concerns raised in online communities could better help care providers address mothers' concerns and fears when it comes to vaccines and medical care more generally.

Finally, a brief comment is needed on the prevalence of health-related narratives in online spaces. The sheer volume of health-related posts in the groups of interest (approximately 50 per cent of posts) is an important data point in itself. This reflects a situation in which mothers feel compelled to look to their peers for advice and information rather than professionals. The compulsion to seek out information, advice, and support from "random people on the internet" may be symptomatic of the pressures and anxieties faced by mothers as they try to take back "a bit of control" (MacKendrick 327). In fact, the act of seeking out communities online may itself be a contemporary manifestation of intensive mothering.

As our social lives become increasingly embedded in digital worlds, medical scholars have an imperative to understand the nature of these social interactions and their impact on people's offline decisions, particularly when it comes to health. We might consider learning more about the draws of such spaces—such as empathy, kindness, ease of access, and the denunciation of sexism, racism, and fatphobia—and consider how medical professionals can continue to emphasize these attributes in their practice.

Endnotes

1. It should be noted that although science and nature are not truly oppositional, the tendency for public and policy framings to conflate them as dichotomous (for example, around discussions of vaccination, breastfeeding, and genetically modified organisms) provides a useful starting point for examining the diversity among perspectives on health and medicine (Brunson and Sobo).

2. "Woo" is a colloquial term for pseudoscience or pseudoscientific.

Works Cited

Audrain-Pontevia, Anne-Francoise, and Loick Menvielle. "Do Online Health Communities Enhance Patient–Physician Relationship? An Assessment of the Impact of Social Support and Patient Empowerment." *Health Services Management Research*, vol. 31, no. 3, 2017, pp. 154-62.

Bird, Chloe E. and Patricia P. Rieker. *Gender and Health*. Cambridge University Press, 2008.

Brunson, Emily K. and Elisa J. Sobo. "Framing Childhood Vaccination in the United States: Getting Past Polarization in the Public Discourse." *Human Organization*, vol. 76, no. 1, 2017, pp. 38-47.

Canizares, Mayilee et al. "Changes in the Use of Practitioner-Based Complementary and Alternative Medicine Over Time in Canada: Cohort and Period Effects." *PLoS One*, vol. 12, no. 5, 2017, p. e0177307–17.

Hardey, Michael. "Doctor in the House: The Internet as a Source of Lay Health Knowledge and the Challenge to Expertise." *Sociology of Health & Illness*, vol. 21, no. 6, 1999, pp. 820-35.

Hays, Sharon. *The Cultural Contradictions of Motherhood*. Yale University Press, 1998.

Holmes, Ryan. "Are Facebook Groups the Future of Social Media (or a Dead End)?" *Forbes*, 29 Oct. 2018, www.forbes.com/sites/ryanholmes/2018/10/29/are-facebook-groups-the-future-of-social-media-or-a-dead-end/?sh=6f7cfc6a1d23. Accessed 27 Mar. 2021.

Kivits, Joëlle. "Everyday Health and the Internet: A Mediated Health Perspective on Health Information Seeking." *Sociology of Health & Illness*, vol. 31, no. 5, 2009, pp. 673-87.

Larsson, Margareta. "A Descriptive Study of the Use of the Internet by Women Seeking Pregnancy-Related Information." *Midwifery*, vol. 25, no. 1, 2009, pp. 14-20.

Lemire, Marc et al. "Determinants of Internet Use as a Preferred Source of Information on Personal Health." *International Journal of Medical Informatics*, vol. 77, no. 11, 2008, pp. 723-34.

Lupton, Deborah. "Consumerism, Reflexivity and the Medical Encounter." *Social Science & Medicine*, vol. 45, no. 3, 1997, pp. 373-81.

MacKendrick, Norah, and Lindsay M. Stevens. "'Taking Back a Little Bit of Control': Managing the Contaminated Body Through Consumption." *Sociological Forum*, vol. 31, no. 2, 2016, pp. 310-29.

Rainie, Lee. "E-Patients and Their Hunt for Health Information." *Pew Research Centre*, 9 Oct. 2013, www.slideshare.net/PewInternet/2013-7-26-13-rise-of-epatients-medical-librarians-la-jolla-pdf. Accessed 27 Mar. 2021.

Reich, Jennifer A. *Calling the Shots*. New York University Press, 2016.

Smith, Naomi, and Tim Graham. "Mapping the Anti-Vaccination Movement on Facebook." *Information, Communication & Society*, vol. 22, no. 9, 2017, pp. 1310-27.

Statistics Canada. "Getting a Second Opinion: Health Information and the Internet." *Statistics Canada*, 7 July 2015, www150.statcan.gc.ca/n1/pub/82-003-x/2008001/article/10515/5002590-eng.htm. Accessed 27 Mar. 2021.

Villalobos, Ana. *Motherload: Making It All Better in Insecure Times*. University of California Press, 2014.

Wodak, Ruth, and Michael Meyer. *Methods of Critical Discourse Analysis*. Sage Publications Ltd, 2001.

Wolf, Joan B. *Is Breast Best?* New York University Press, 2013.

Zaslow, Emilie. "Revalorizing Feminine Ways of Knowing." *Information, Communication & Society*, vol. 15, no. 9, 2012, pp. 1352-72.

Chapter 13

Sha-reer (Body), Ka-mee (Deficiency), and Kum-joa-ree (Weakness): Articulations and Interpretations of Pregnancy and Childbirth in a Marginalized Community in India

Alekhya "Baba" Das

Introduction and Theoretical Framework

This chapter examines women's agency and autonomy in their articulations and interpretations about not only pregnancy regimes and birthing but also their postnatal bodily experiences and perceptions concerning women's illness, deficiencies, and wellbeing. The objective is to address the following question: Do socially, culturally, and economically marginalized women have agency and autonomy, especially as regards their reproductive health and bodies? Moreover, how does one locate and comprehend this agency and autonomy? This chapter derives from the author's research (conducting in 2009 and 2010) regarding the role of husbands as well as marital relations in the health-seeking behaviour of impoverished and marginalized women living in the slum neighbourhood of Gautampuri in Delhi, India.

A qualitative design and fieldwork strategy were employed for this study, using ethnographic and participant observation methods. In addition, semistructured interviews and focus groups were conducted with women and men (n=12 each) and with community workers (n=10). The primary data were collected in Hindi-Urdu language and were then translated and transcribed into English and analyzed using discourse, narrative, and content analyses. The University of New Brunswick's (Fredericton, NB, Canada) research ethics procedures were followed, and, accordingly, all of the participants were given pseudonyms. The data provided in this chapter originate from focus group discussions with women and men (cited as "FGW" and "FGM," respectively) as well as from field notes.

Critical and phenomenological feminist theory frame this chapter. The different waves of feminism have helped to emphasize women's autonomy and agency, given that "a woman's life depends upon an exercise of bodily autonomy and on social conditions that enable that autonomy" (Butler, *Undoing Gender* 12). Linking lived experience and agency, Butler further argues that a cultural construction "is not opposed to agency; it is the necessary scene of agency, the very terms in which agency is articulated and becomes culturally intelligible" (*Gender Trouble*, 201).

Among the authors and scholars who build on these theoretical frameworks, many also concentrate on women's bodies, women's illnesses and wellbeing, gender and healthcare delivery, and institutionalized medical care. Since "our lived experience is inflected by gender and sexual difference, illness experiences are highly conditioned by gender [and] are manifestly always already gendered on the existential and empirical level" (Fisher 28). This chapter expands on this body of literature, which critiques privileging expert-defined reproductive health and wellbeing over interpretative definitions of pregnancy, childbirth, and sexuality (Käll and Zeiler 1-2; Fisher 28). Other similar studies critically assess medico-scientific and insti-tutionalized discourses as well as the absence of women's agency and narratives about their bodies, ailments, and wellbeing in research designs and outcomes (Fisher 33; McLeod 1; Adams and Burcher 74).

Background

Biomedical awareness about women's diseases and their causes is largely absent in this community in Delhi, and my informants have limited clinical knowledge about human anatomy and the biochemical causes behind various bodily phenomena (such as fevers or menstruation). Women's health-seeking behavior in this community pertains to using professional medical care (for both ailments and reproductive concerns). At a broader level, their health-seeking behaviour includes behaviours towards overall wellbeing as well as preventing illnesses and bodily harms. Various factors, such as definitions of what is healthy and unhealthy or not, considerably shape women's health-seeking behaviour, including for reproductive matters. In order to analyse these women's reproductive health-seeking behaviour, it is necessary to comprehend their "rhetoric of yesteryears." During focus groups and interviews, I observed a pattern within the narratives in which the informants privileged their life in the past. For instance, informants frequently discussed how they had superior lives in the past, along with their family, community, and environment.

Bodies, Deficiencies, Wellbeing, and Illnesses

In this community, women's health-seeking behaviour regarding reproduction comprises pregnancy, childbirth, and postnatal behaviours. These behaviours, in turn, are shaped by other segments of their health-seeking behaviour, such as beliefs regarding women's bodies, definitions of healthy and unhealthy, and interpretations of diseases. Perceptions concerning the body are central to the definitions and interpretations of women's illnesses, which are articulated by using three categories: the body (sha-reer), bodily sensations (such as durd [pain]), and bodily experiences (such as feeling a-jeeb [uncanny] about their bodies).

The physical body (sha-reer) may refer to the outside or surface of the body as well as to the body's interior (such as internal organs, blood, and so on). As per these women, there is a compelling connection between their physical body and the ailments they have or may obtain later. Moreover, certain women's illnesses originate from the physical body. The second category comprises narratives about bodily sensations, such as aches and pains, such as kam-ur durd (backache), see-nay may durd (chest pain), and ba-chay daa-nee may soo-jun (soreness in vaginal area). The third category concerns experiencing peculiar sensations, feeling unsure about their bodies, and generally lacking bodily control, such as bay-chain-ee (restlessness), chak-kur (giddiness), and ghab-raa-hut (panicky). These women also connect the sha-reer (body), kum-joaree (weakness), and ka-mee (deficiency) in the body. They believe that women can be born with bodily deficiency or acquire deficiency through improper nutrition, and this bodily deficiency is connected to several ailments. Moreover, deficiencies can be corrected through replenishing their bodies with proper nutrition, such as with traditional foods.

In this community, women's wellbeing is defined through physical mobility and the ability to perform household tasks. Conversely, illness or a state of ailing or feeling unhealthy is signified by immobility and a woman's inability to perform day-to-day errands. Moreover, immobility is a more important facet while defining women's health, as this community deems almost all bodily states as "healthy" as long as there is no sign of immobility in the woman—a mobile body is a healthy body. This community defines illnesses and ailments by using two dualities. The first is baa-ha-ree (external) versus un-droo-nee (internal) bee-maa-ree (ailments). External ailments have externally perceptible symptoms (such as a visible wound), whereas internal ailments originate inside the body (such as ulcers or tumors). To be detected, internal ailments require the work of trained doctors who use complex technology (like X-Ray machines) to "look inside" the body; hence, residents tend to take internal ailments more seriously. The second duality is maa-moo-lee (minor) versus ba-dee (major) ailments. Pain in joa-day (joints) is a recurrent example of a minor ailment, whereas an ailment that necessitates hospitalization is a major illness.

Bodily otherness, or having an uncanny body, as reported in my study, is also a recurring theme within feminist literature about women's health. Anorexia, dysmorphic body perceptions, body image, and plastic/augmentative surgery are all instances of women negotiating control (or lack of control) over their bodies. Numerous feminist studies have noted how pregnant women can often experience their bodies as foreign as well as have postnatal desires to restore their bodies to their prepregnancy form though diet, starving, exercise, surgery, or medication (McLeod 133-34; Svenaeus 201). Consequently, many feminist scholars situate reproduction, maternity, pregnancy and wellbeing, within "analyses of issues such as bodily self-experience, normality and deviance, self-alienation and objectification" (Käll and Zeiler 2).

Pregnancies, Precautions, and Potent/Impotent Bodies

Many of this community's discourses regarding pregnancy involve beliefs about proper foods and nutrition for pregnant women:

> Put some mashed sub-jee [vegetables], extra la-soon [garlic] and mir-chee [green pepper] in the stuffed roa-tee [flatbread]. That helps [to build up strength of pregnant women]. (Kangna, FGW)

> I fed her [pregnant wife] ghee [clarified butter] and baa-daam [almonds]. I bought kish-mish [raisins] ... first of all these things are necessary [during pregnancy] ... then ad-rak [ginger], hull-dee [powdered turmeric], doodh [milk]. (Mool Chand, FGM)

Similarly, there are several narratives about appropriate prenatal behaviours and precautions: "Well, I took take some rest indoors [before delivery] ... an expectant woman should not suddenly get up and run around; she may catch ha-waa [wind/ 'bad' air]" (Shabana, FGW). Shabana, like many members of this community, believes that wind or air causes many health problems. Hence, pregnant women should be additionally careful because they are particularly vulnerable to bad winds, which may affect their health or harm the baby.

The "rhetoric of yesteryears" is important for comprehending women's pregnancy practices in this community. For instance, with reference to prenatal medical care, informants said that it was inconsequential in their past. Due to the past's "purer" environment, women in their community were born with "pure" bodies. Hence, the very constitution of women's bodies was potent from birth as well as superior to that of the current generation. This kind of pure and potent body was almost immune to every possible ailment and was capable of functioning without any professional medical help, such as during childbirth. For this reason, many wives asserted that in the past, pregnant women in their community did not require any of the modern-day prenatal tests and medical checkups: "No, we did not avail them, none of these things [prenatal checkups and tests/vaccinations]" (Hema, FGW). These wives claim that unlike the present, women in the past

155

had sound sha-reer (physiques); consequently, even without these prenatal medical regimes, they coped with pregnancy and gave birth without any problem. Informants further explained that owing to the "impure" character of the present times, women in their community are no longer born with pure bodies. Instead, nowadays women are born with bodies containing several ka-mee (deficiencies), which is why women of the current generation require all forms of external interventions, such as prenatal checkups, assistance from reproductive healthcare professionals, vaccinations, and supplements.

Other informants believed that their past was significantly dissimilar to the present, since nowadays their community has a propensity to seek medical care even for minor health issues. As a result, pregnancies are becoming overly dependent on institutional medical care. As Susheela said, "Earlier we [women and community members in general] never used to visit a doctor unless it was extremely necessary ... nowadays women go to the doctor even for smallest of ailment" (FGW). The informants said that professional medicine does not have the same importance as traditional diet or women's bodily construction within the pregnancy or childbirth-related regimes in this community, which is why it did not historically feature in the reproductive behaviours of these women. Although prenatal immunisations were readily available in the past, few had access to them.

Eating appropriate food during pregnancy is also important for marginalized groups in India, such as "special foods that they had brought from the village: flours of roasted chickpea and barley, rice from one's family fields, pickle (achar) of hand-picked mangoes, and clarified butter (ghee)" (Snell-Rood 283). Other studies reveal precautions some pregnant women take, such as "rituals to follow during pregnancy," such as "never sitting in the traditional Indian cross-legged position" or sleeping on their back (Corbett and Callister 301). In addition, bodily beliefs interpreted via the "rhetoric of yesteryears" are also prevalent among the slum populations of Delhi, since with reference to women, "certain aspects of the body were determined at birth" (Snell-Rood 281).

Postpartum and Birthing Bodies

How ailments are defined also shape beliefs about childbirth, which is perceived as mystifying and worrisome, since childbirth concerns the interior of a woman's body and is, thus, comparable to an internal ailment (as explained previously). The definitions of "wellbeing" (signified by mobility) and "unwell" (signified by immobility) also shape women's beliefs and behaviours regarding pregnancy, birthing, and the postpartum phase. To illustrate, my informants talked about the prenatal and postnatal phases as unexceptional and routine aspects of their lives. Thus, many wives recollected their experiences with indifference:

> [I did] Everything [household chores] on my own. I had my baby in the morning, by evening I was sweeping, washing ... [very dispassionate tone], also bathing the child, cleaning him, drying him, putting him to sleep. (Aarti, FGW)

> [For delivery] I go to my natal home in ... my village ... last time when I was pregnant, I took the train today, I reached tomorrow and I gave birth the day after, took [the] train, and returned. [matter of factly speaking manner] (Kangna, FGW)

Based on the aforementioned responses, it is clear that pregnant women in this community remain mobile and continue to do their daily chores due to the fact that pregnancy is perceived within the realm of health and wellbeing. A sense of unwellness denotes aberration or abnormality, whereas for this community, pregnancy is anything but abnormal or unusual.

For this reason, these women are reluctant to seek institutional delivery, as hospitals are for major ailments, which is contrary to their perception of birthing. Consequently, informants find it perplexing that government agencies, healthcare establishments, and Arpana (a community organisation) all portray pregnancy as something extraordinary, which needs dedicated care from other family members and specialized attention from trained healthcare professionals. Therefore, when I asked these women who was caring for them during their advanced pregnancy, I only received counter questions, such as "Why should anyone take care of pregnant women?" or "Is pregnancy a sickness?" These questions highlighted the strangeness of my question vis-à-vis comparing pregnancy and sickness, given that my question conflicted with their collectively held beliefs about giving birth.

Past research has unearthed similar perceptions among marginalized communities in India regarding prenatal, birthing, and postnatal practices. For example, some daughters-in-law are asked to carry on or do more domestic chores, as that will maintain the flexibility of the body, thereby aiding natural childbirth (Corbett and Callister 301-02; Moursund and Kravdal 285-87). Furthermore, in some slums in India, "70% of women with neonatal deaths thought that it was not customary or necessary to have antenatal care or safe delivery" (Ghosh and Sharma 526)—an observation that is supported by this study. Researchers have found similar narratives surrounding reproductive health among marginalized women in Bangladesh, where women subscribe to both to the "juxtaposition of folk and biomedical explanations" as well as to medical beliefs consisting of "notions about food, sexuality, bodily beliefs, marital situation and poverty" (Rashid 111).

Discussion and Conclusion

Structures of domination and constraints exist in multiple domains for marginalized women, in the India subcontinent. Women in marginalized communities in India experience power imbalances within domestic and social structures, which intersect with institutional contexts, such as medical care regimes, healthcare establishments, health professionals, and service providers. So, do these women display agency regarding their bodies, birthing as well as their pregnancy experiences? As this study shows, and despite the aforementioned structural constraints, women do express their agency and autonomy, which are both explicit and tacit. The choices these women make regarding their pregnant bodies, prenatal life experiences, childbirth traditions, and postnatal behaviors broadly affirm their agency, as they assert control over at least their reproductive health, including their preferred cures and treatments.

However, the agentic actions, narratives, and discourses of marginalized women are typically neglected by most theoretical frameworks and disciplines—notably public health, health sciences, healthcare management, and social work—since they privilege institutional discourses and narratives of authority. In addition, these narratives are rarely featured in research; thus, these women's lived experiences and agency become invisible and deemed nonexistent. In order to shed light on these women's agency and autonomy, this chapter applies feminist and phenomenological theoretical frameworks because it is vital to focus on the uniqueness of lived experiences of the marginalized, oppressed, and socially invisible. By raising highlighting experiences of sexuality, pregnancy, and birth, feminism and phenomenological schools have noted the importance of embodiment and situatedness in uncovering the meaning of illness for different communities (Käll and Zeiler 2; Butler, Undoing Gender 12; McLeod 1-2).

Objectivist research, often embedded with patriarchal dispositions of healthcare in the Indian subcontinent, presumes and depicts women as passive, unaware, and powerless regarding their bodies, reproduction, health, and illnesses (Moursund and Kravdal 285-86). This study critiques these presumptions and conclusions and reveals that women's actions surrounding pregnancy and giving birth—including the use of collective knowledge, such as concrete definitions about bodies as well as categorizations of physical environments—make coherent the interconnections between observed symptoms in bodies and probable causes (for example wind and bodily deficiencies). This study demonstrates the importance of women's and subjectivist perspectives regarding their understanding of birth and maternity. The emphasis on the pertinence of feminist and phenomenological frameworks is substantiated by scholars studying urban poor in the Indian subcontinent, given that women make links among poverty, tension, everyday worries in order to explain bodily occurrences like white discharges. Narratives about "weakness" and "worry illnesses" are "metaphors for the economic, social, and political deprivation in poor women's lives" (Rashid 111). Therefore, urban poor women's own understanding of their reproductive experiences must be highlighted, since they significantly diverge from biomedical and institutional explanations.

Also evident from this study is these women's ability to act and think refelxively regarding being healthy and having "normal" bodies as well as identifying ailing and "abnormal" bodies; they also critically question powerful voices (such as healthcare professionals as well as government officials) when their message conflicts with these women's own beliefs, which troubles the common portrayal of these women as passive. Feminist studies about how women often feel they lose control over their own body during pregnancy and childbirth show that "women's bodily self-alienation comes to articulation at intersections of different categories of identity and structures of power and privilege" (McLeod 1). Physicians and nurses assuming control of the birthing body is, thus, an example of bodily alienation (Adams and Burcher 8). The conclusions of this study, therefore, augment a section of feminist literature, which asserts that bodily subjectivities and experiences provide a site for critical and feminist examination of antenatal and postnatal care, childbirth regimes and practices, as well as the agency of pregnant women and mothers (Käll and Zeiler 2).

Works Cited

Adams, Sarah L., and Paul Burcher. "Communal Pushing: Childbirth and Intersubjectivity." *Feminist Phenomenology and Medicine*, edited by Lisa F. Kall and Kristin Zeiler, State University of New York Press, 2014, pp. 69-80.

Butler, Judith, and Elizabeth Weed. *The Question of Gender: Joan W. Scott's Critical Feminism*. Indiana University Press, 2011.

Butler, Judith. *Gender Trouble: Feminism and the Subversion of Identity*. Routledge, 2007.

Butler, Judith. *Undoing Gender*. Routledge, 2004.

Chattopadhyay, Aparajita. "Men in Maternal Care: Evidence from India." *J Biosoc Sci.*, vol. 44, no. 2, 2012, pp. 129-53.

Corbett, Cheryl A., and Lynn C. Callister. "Giving Birth: The Voices of Women in Tamil Nadu, India." *The American Journal of Maternal/Child Nursing*, vol. 37, no. 5, 2012, pp. 298-305.

Fisher, Linda. "The Illness Experience: A Feminist Phenomenological Perspective." *Feminist Phenomenology and Medicine*, edited by Lisa. F. Kall and Kristin Zeiler, State University of New York Press, 2014, pp. 27-46.

Kall, Lisa F., and Kristin Zeiler. "Why Feminist Phenomenology and Medicine?" *Feminist Phenomenology and Medicine*, edited by Lisa F. Kall and Kristin Zeiler, State University of New York Press, 2014, pp. 1-26.

McLeod, Carolyn. *Self-Trust and Reproductive Autonomy*. The MIT Press, 2002.

Moursund, Anne, and Oystein Kravdal. "Individual and Community Effects of Women's Education and Autonomy on Contraceptive Use in India." *Population Studies*, vol. 57, no. 3, 2003, pp. 285-301.

Mullany, Britta C., et al. "Can Women's Autonomy Impede Male Involvement in Pregnancy Health in Katmandu, Nepal?" *Social Science & Medicine*, vol. 61, no. 9, 2005, pp. 1993-2006.

Mumtaz, Zubia, and Sarah Salway. "Understanding Gendered Influences on Women's Reproductive Health in Pakistan: Moving beyond the Autonomy Paradigm." *Social Science & Medicine,* vol. 68, no. 7, 2009, pp. 1349-56.

Nahar, Papreen. "Health Seeking Behaviour of Childless Women in Bangladesh: An Ethnographic Exploration for the Special Issue On—Loss in Child bearing." *Social Science & Medicine*, vol. 71, no. 10, 2010, pp. 1780-87.

Rashid, Sabina F. "Durbolota (Weakness), Chinta Rog (Worry Illness), and Poverty Explanations of White Discharge among Married Adolescent Women in an Urban Slum in Dhaka, Bangladesh." *Medical Anthropology Quarterly*, vol. 21, no. 1, 2007, pp. 108-32.

Saikia, Nandita, and Abhishek Singh. "Does Type of Household Affect Maternal Health? Evidence from India." *J Biosoc Sci.*, vol. 41, no. 3, 2009, pp. 329-53.

Snell-Rood, Claire. "To Know the Field: Shaping the Slum Environment and Cultivating the Self." *ETHOS*, vol. 41, no. 3, 2013, pp. 271-91.

Svenaeus, Fredrik. "The Body Uncanny: Alienation, Illness, and Anorexia Nervosa." *Feminist Phenomenology and Medicine*, edited by Lisa F. Kall and Kristin Zeiler, State University of New York Press, 2014, pp. 201-22.

Chapter 14

"There's Just Not Enough Out There": The Role of Scarcity in Framing Postpartum Depression

Hannah Rochelle Davidson

> As many women explained, I was the first person to express an interest in, and explicitly ask them about, an aspect of their lives they felt was silenced and condemned by society and the people around them.
>
> —Natasha Mauthner (90)

Claims of scarcity permeate the literature—academic, personal, popular, and organizational—on postpartum depression. In my day-to-day life, I hear about aunts, mothers, sisters, cousins, and friends who suffer from postpartum depression and feel a scarcity of resources, of support, or of visibility of the disorder itself. Whether it is an academic trying to critically situate postpartum depression, a mother articulating her narrative of the disorder, or an organization trying to clarify the finer details of what postpartum depression is and is not, the scarcity takes many forms.

In contrast to this dominant claim, my research on postpartum depression's clinical life has revealed a history that is anything but scarce. The desire to build knowledge about postpartum depression has inspired countless research institutes, clinical investigations, community-based interventions, nonprofits, helplines, blog posts, and academic books and anthologies. Desire to spread awareness about postpartum depression in the contemporary sphere has also inspired numerous celebrity memoirs and media plotlines. These voices clamour for amplification, often trying desperately to act against a presupposed scarcity.

The purpose of this chapter is to complicate the idea of scarcity in claims about postpartum depression by presenting a new working history of the condition itself. Following this working history, this chapter examines the ways in which the scarcity claim is enacted in modern clinical care through the findings in my interviews with care providers. Together, the history and voices of these actors in maternal healthcare illuminate inherent dualities in the existing claims on postpartum depression. Quickly, postpartum depression transforms from a relatively young diagnosable condition into a disorder that is both viscerally and historically seen and felt yet is also not seen enough. Locating this duality through the vehicle of scarcity reveals the vital context needed for assessing the cultural, medical, and subjective meanings of postpartum depression as a diagnosis and disorder in the present moment.

Medicalizing Maternal Sadness: Early Accounts of Postpartum Depression

Early psychiatric accounts of female asylum patients describe the existence of puerperal insanity—a condition whose symptoms closely resemble what is presently diagnosed as postpartum depression—as early as the mid-nineteenth century (Freeman et al.). Approximately 10 per cent of asylum patient admissions in the nineteenth century are estimated to have been for puerperal insanity (Freeman et al.; Taylor; Dubriwny), which is often characterized by a constellation of symptoms, including "using obscenity, aversion to the child and her husband, and meanness" (Dubriwny 72). Other accounts describe mothers being taken over by "milk fever"—that is, the coinciding onset of lactation with depressive or irritable symptoms (Freeman et al.).

When and how did an illness whose characteristics have been noted in medical literature since the late nineteenth century begin to be characterized as scarce? Answering this requires an understanding, in broad strokes, of how the mental healthcare industry transformed in the span of a century. Standard care for mothers suffering from puerperal insanity in the late nineteenth century was to withdraw the mother from her community. For some, this meant admittance into asylums; for others, like the protagonist in *The Yellow Wallpaper*, it looked like confinement to the hearth—intellectual activities suspended and subjected to the "resting" cure (*Gilman*, "Why I Wrote The Yellow Wallpaper"). The literal removal of mentally ill women—specifically mothers—from the community at large is connected to modern claims of scarcity projected onto postpartum depression today. By manufacturing scarcity of emotional distress in postpartum, early practices of managing symptoms similar to postpartum depression effectively embedded postpartum depression within a complex web of shame, silence, and stigma.

Feminist Organizing and Foundations of the Modern Postpartum Depression Movement

The shift necessary to change the conversation about postpartum depression would come as social progress and transitions in healthcare created a perfect storm for postpartum advocacy efforts in the latter part of the twentieth century. In *Rock-a-by Baby: Feminism, Self-Help, and Postpartum Depression*, Verta Taylor asserts that the emergence of modern postpartum depression awareness stems from the self-help movement of the 1980s, which in turn spawned an orchestrated postpartum depression awareness campaign. The emergence of contemporary awareness of postpartum depression, Taylor argues, has roots in first-wave feminism, where "it was in the women's health movement that self-help took center stage" (Taylor 63). The women's health movement was the product of an understanding that the dissemination of knowledge around women's health was made a scarce commodity by a hegemonic medical system. Peer groups in the women's health movement functioned by creating informal networks of women that mobilized and recirculated knowledges previously controlled by the biomedical sphere (Morgen). However, these early knowledge projects did little to acknowledge the possibility of emotional distress after giving birth. In fact, as Taylor elaborates, her field work of interviewing women involved in the creation of "Our Bodies,

Ourselves" illuminated how the very little bit of acknowledgment given to postpartum depression existed in the final work almost by chance:

> A collective member ... recalled a woman she described as "very thin, almost waify, and not very vivacious who kept bringing up postpartum depression".... [She] remembered thinking, like most other members of the mostly college-age group, that "postpartum depression didn't seem very interesting or important and that this woman was probably off on her own hysterical little thing, that this problem just didn't seem central to the women's movement." But she quickly added that "the way the women's movement functioned in its early stages was that the problems it dealt with came entirely out of women's own experiences, so this woman, nevertheless, ended up writing a section on postpartum depression for the book." (67)

As this passage indicates, postpartum depression was not handled with the magnitude of other reproductive health themes at the outset of the women's health movement. Instead, those voices most integral to the early women's health movement struggled to take postpartum depression seriously, handling the condition with the same patriarchal attitudes reserved for other women's psychiatric disorders. Still, the mere acknowledgment of postpartum depression within these circles set in place a movement peripheral to the women's health movement but with different motivations and objectives.

Whereas the women's health movement sought to democratize information about reproductive health, peer-based organizing around postpartum depression centred around breaking silences, thus making emotional distress in postpartum visible. This desire for visibility and breaking silence also affected the objectives of this sort of peer organizing. The women's health movement operated parallel to the clinic, including the dissemination of information in peer groups and through peer-designed publication, whereas organizing around postpartum depression ultimately focused on the clinical recognition of postpartum depression and associated perinatal mental health disorders. The combination of these movements made the early postpartum depression awareness most amenable to the formation of peer-based support groups, where women came together to articulate their emotional suffering experienced after birth. This peer support group model is a pivotal one, which ultimately transformed community-based support for postpartum depression, with many support groups still actively running across the United States (US) today (Dennis).

Towards a Clinical Recognition of Postpartum Depression

As the discourse grew to resemble a concerted movement towards postpartum depression awareness, several key figures and actions coalesced to solidify postpartum depression's present status as legitimate condition. In 1980, the Marcé Society for Perinatal Mental Health was founded in the United Kingdom. Named after Louis Victor Marcé, one of the first physicians to describe puerperal mental illness in the nineteenth century, the society's intention was to create an international and interdisciplinary professional society entirely devoted to what they described chiefly as postnatal mental illness (Glangeaud). This society was the child of several professionals working in perinatal mental health, who were interested in gathering together professionals in various fields—including medicine, allied health, and academia—to convene and share knowledge ("History").

With intellectual scaffolding came an influx of organizational development. In 1985, Depression After Delivery (DAD), one of the first advocacy organizations specifically aimed at supporting mothers with postpartum depression in the US, was formed (Taylor). In 1987, Jane Honikman formed Postpartum Support International (PSI), which is still in operation today. PSI was founded with the intent of "promoting awareness, prevention, and treatment" of postpartum depression and has grown to encompass various peer and professional advocacy, training, and support structures ("About PSI—Overview").

Modern Accounts of the Scarcity Claim

What function does scarcity serve in the modern maternal mental healthcare system or in the ways that mothers, care providers, and other mental health workers make sense of postpartum depression? This section argues for the continued existence of a scarcity claim in the contemporary life of postpartum depression and that this claim has several functions. First, it is indicative of gaps that persist because of the shaky, decades-long transition from institutional to community-based mental healthcare. Scarcity in a contemporary professional context often translates to a lack of institutional resources and education for providers.

Providing Care and Coming to Know Postpartum Depression

When asked what exposure the care providers I interviewed had to postpartum depression before practicing medicine, many of my interlocutors came up short. Some had intimate knowledge or preexisting interest in postpartum depression. Others admitted that they knew very little or that the knowledge they did develop about postpartum depression came from a few select interactions early on in their career. I found these stories from providers compelling, not only because they revealed a sort of humility and honesty from the providers themselves but also because they made clear the ways in which for many individuals—even skilled providers—postpartum depression, like the postpartum experience, is not on the forefront of every person's mind.

Medical education in the US is considered rigorous and culturally perceived as all-encompassing: this, in part, contributes to the cultural capital held by physicians (Wagner). However, postpartum depression treatment is lacking in physician training and education, particularly for obstetric, paediatric, and other primary care providers (Wisner et al.). Said Brenda, a psychiatrist working in New York City:

> We need to provide better training and resources to the OB/ GYNs because I think many of them are just too scared to even ask the questions ... and—so they don't ask mental health questions because they really don't know what to do once they get someone who tells them they do in fact have mental illness symptoms ... they're totally overwhelmed. So, they avoid asking. And ... that's a huge part of the problem.

This lack of education about postpartum depression in medical training is reflective of a general scarcity in mental health training for primary care providers. This lack of circulating knowledge—even though, as my research indicates, resources do exist to adequately train and inform providers—creates a manufactured scarcity, where the problem of postpartum depression most certainly exists, but providers are not trained to adequately, as one physician described it to me, "sniff it out."

Health Insurance, Mental Health Cost, and the Maintenance of Scarcity

The power of health insurance in healthcare in the US has grown greatly in the post-WWII era. In 1940, fewer than 10 per cent of the US population had health insurance (Weisbrod); in 2017, the number was closer to 92 per cent (US Census Bureau). The shift to an insurance-reimbursed care system, alongside the growth and emphasis of medical technologies, has contributed to an emphasis on a technocratic model of care that prioritizes the use of advanced medical technology over traditional or less technologically advanced modes of enacting care (Davis-Floyd).

The complex transformation on systems of care enacted by the shift to an insurance-based model of health expense compensation increased the national spending on healthcare significantly (Weisbrod). The one form of healthcare expense that did not increase over the same span of time, however, was the spending in mental healthcare (Frank and Glied). Some of this stabilizing in mental healthcare spending was actually due in part to the efficiency of certain health technologies, including the emergence of managed behavioural health organizations (MBHOs), the ways in which Medicare spending captures a fraction of mental healthcare for those most vulnerable in the population, and the emergence of new pharmaceutical management techniques for specific mental illnesses, such as bipolar disorder and schizophrenia (Frank and Glied).

While these technologies, coupled with the dominating force of insurance in healthcare, stabilized certain mental healthcare structures, they also made scarce certain ways of enacting care in mental health. Talk therapy, for instance, is still poorly reimbursed for psychiatrists—a fact that several physicians emphasized in their interviews and best summarized by family physician Alison's remark: "I can't believe how little psychiatrists get paid. It's worse than paediatrics, as far as that. And they can't double book or do procedures; they're just kind of stuck."

In a system where health insurance reimbursement for services ultimately controls *how* and for what price services providers are compensated, certain services will be prioritized over others. Prevailing models of insurance reimbursement prioritize the ability to, as Alison describes, "double book" appointments, which is often challenging or impossible to do when providing talk therapy. These forces, shaped by the priorities of insurance companies themselves, make certain modes of care inaccessible to providers, who may in theory want to provide the best care possible to their patients yet in practice still need to adhere to enacting care under a capitalist system.

The priorities and structures of insurance reimbursement, then, reify the scarcity of the condition by preventing the conversation about postpartum depression from happening in the first place. For example, the very skills required to bring visibility to postpartum depression— taking the time to screen a mother and then consult her about her various options—are not incentivized via insurance, nor do they fit in a specific billable category for most of the providers that provide care to people in the postpartum period. Talking, after all, is not a new technology that can be readily monetized. This reality was emphasized by several of the providers I interviewed:

> Christine: Right now, [screening for postpartum depression is] not reimbursed. So it would be helpful if prevention was reimbursed properly ... via healthcare, via the health plan. So, somebody—well, [in Massachusetts] ... the providers do get reimbursed for our publicly insured patients ... once in pregnancy and once in postpartum. But in most of the places, it's not reimbursed. So you're adding an extra task onto these pro-viders—that is, you know, that they don't get paid for.

> Brenda: And [primary care providers] aren't talking to their patients because, again, insurance companies aren't reimbursing them for their time to talk to patients. So, you know, while I'm not an antimedication ... by any means, many people do not need to be on medication, and they would do well with the talk therapy.... And primary care doctors— ... who are on insurance plans—can't afford to sit and talk to patients. And so, that's another way that people are getting, you know, tremendously underserved—by only getting pharmacology and not getting talk therapy.

Although Christine and Brenda work in different states with different dynamics of insurance reimbursement, they both point to the vast scarcity of incentive for postpartum depression screening and care from the perspective of insurance care. Although there has been some progress in addressing this scarcity—Alison, the family physician I spoke with, explained that the Affordable Care Act increased the insurance reimbursement amount for psychiatrists by state insurance—there is still much progress to be made in terms of addressing the scarcity manufactured by systemic powers, especially in terms of health insurance and medical education.

Works Cited

"About PSI—Overview." *Postpartum Support—PSI*, www.postpartum. net/about-psi/overview/. Accessed 16 Apr. 2019.

US Census Bureau. *Health Insurance Coverage in the United States: 2017, Census,* 2017, www.census.gov/library/publications/2018/demo/ p60-264.html. Accessed 27 Mar. 2021.

Davis-Floyd, R. "The Technocratic, Humanistic, and Holistic Paradigms of Childbirth." *International Journal of Gynaecology and Obstetrics: The Official Organ of the International Federation of Gynaecology and Obstetrics*, vol. 75 Suppl 1, Nov. 2001, pp. S5-23.

Dennis, Cindy-Lee. "Postpartum Depression Peer Support: Maternal Perceptions from a Randomized Controlled Trial." *International Journal of Nursing Studies*, vol. 47, no. 5, May 2010, pp. 560-68. *ScienceDirect*, doi:10.1016/j.ijnurstu.2009.10.015.

Dubriwny, Tasha N., editor. "Postfeminist Risky Mothers and Postpartum Depression." *The Vulnerable Empowered Woman*, Rutgers University Press, edited by Tasha N. Dubriwny, 2013, pp. 69-106, / www.jstor.org.5colauthen.library.umass.edu/stable/j.ctt5hjfnz.7.

Frank, Richard G., and Sherry Glied. "Changes In Mental Health Financing Since 1971: Implications for Policymakers And Patients." *Health Affairs*, vol. 25, no. 3, 2006, pp. 601-13.

Freeman, Phyllis R., et al. "Margery Kempe, a New Theory: The Inadequacy of Hysteria and Postpartum Psychosis as Diagnostic Categories." *History of Psychiatry*, vol. 1, no. 2, June 1990, pp. 169-90. *SAGE Journals*, doi:10.1177/0957154X9000100202.

Gilman, Sander, and John Conolly. *The Face of Madness: Hugh W. Diamond and the Origin of Psychiatric Photography.* Echo Point Books and Media, 2015.

Gilman, Charlotte Perkins. "Why I Wrote The Yellow Wallpaper." *Cuny,* www.americanyawp.com/reader/18-industrial-america/charlotte-perkins-gilman-why-i-wrote-the-yellow-wallpaper-1913/. Accessed 26 Sept. 2018.

Goffman, Erving. "On the Characteristics of Total Institutions." *Asylums: Essays on the Social Situation of Mental Patients and Other Inmates,* edited by Erving Goffman, Anchor Books, Doubleday & Company, Inc., 1961, pp. 1-67.

"History." *The International Marcé Society for Perinatal Mental Health,* 2021, marcesociety.com/about/history/. Accessed 27 Mar. 2021.

Kerker, Bonnie D., et al. "Identifying Maternal Depression in Pediatric Primary Care: Changes over a Decade." *Journal of Developmental and Behavioral Pediatrics : JDBP,* vol. 37, no. 2, 2016, pp. 113-20. *PubMed Central,* doi:10.1097/DBP.0000000000000255.

Kritsotaki, Despo, et al. *Deinstitutionalisation and After: Post-War Psychiatry in the Western World.* Springer, 2016.

Mauthner, Natasha. "Imprisoned in My Own Prison: A Relational Understanding of Sonya's Story of Postpartum Depression". *Situating Sadness: Women and Depression in Social Context,* edited by Janet M. Stoppard and Linda M. McMullen, New York University Press, 2003, pp. 87-112.

Morgen, Sandra. *Into Our Own Hands: The Women's Health Movement in the United States, 1969–1990.* Rutgers University Press, 2002.

Nicolson, Paula. "Postpartum Depression: Women's Accounts of Loss and Change." *Situating Sadness: Women and Depression in Social Context,* edited by Janet M. Stoppard and Linda M. McMullen, New York University Press, 2003, pp. 113-140.

Novella, Enric J. "Mental Health Care and the Politics of Inclusion: A Social Systems Account of Psychiatric Deinstitutionalization." *Theoretical Medicine and Bioethics,* vol. 31, no. 6, Dec. 2010, pp. 411-27. *Springer Link,* doi:10.1007/s11017-010-9155-8.

Sharpe, Virginia Ashby, et al. *Medical Harm: Historical, Conceptual and Ethical Dimensions of Iatrogenic Illness.* Cambridge University Press, 1998.

Taylor, Verta. *Rock-a-by Baby : Feminism, Self-Help and Postpartum Depression*. Routledge, 2016.

Wagner, Marsden. *Born in the USA: How a Broken Maternity System Must Be Fixed to Put Women and Children First*. University of California Press, 2008.

Weisbrod, Burton A. "The Health Care Quadrilemma: An Essay on Technological Change, Insurance, Quality of Care, and Cost Containment." *Journal of Economic Literature*, vol. 29, no. 2, 1991, pp. 523-52.

Wisner, Katherine L., et al. "Web-Based Education for Postpartum Depression: Conceptual Development and Impact." *Archives of Women's Mental Health*, vol. 11, no. 5, Sept. 2008, p. 377. *Springer Link*, doi:10.1007/s00737-008-0030-9.

Chapter 15

Maternity among Female Physicians in Cameroon: Crossroads between Medical Knowledge and Obstetrical Experience

Jeannette Wogaing

Introduction

Several social scientists have addressed the subject of maternity experience (Jacques "Sociologie de l'accouchement"; Cohen "*Être mère et médecin généraliste*"; Wogaing, "Repenser l'accouchement") and maternal mortality (Wogaing, "*Maternité et décès maternels*"). However, there is a paucity of research in the Cameroonian setting regarding the quest for maternity among female physicians in a country with increasing rates of maternal mortality (782 deaths per 100,000 live births according to the 2011 Demographic and Health Survey).

For a long time, researchers had thought that maternal death concerned only literate or illiterate girls and women residing in rural areas with limited access to quality healthcare facilities and/or personnel. In Cameroon recently, several hospital scandals have overwhelmed the media, including the death of a young physician following complications relating to her pregnancy. This tragedy made us want to better understand how female physicians experience and manage their maternity in such an environment (Boni 166). Does their scientific knowledge in this domain influence their quest for maternity, since they are fully aware of the risks involved?

Method

In a bid to answer this question, we used qualitative research methods. The study took place from December 2018 to February 2019 and involved collecting data on the life stories and maternity experiences of female physicians who had given birth in Cameroonian hospitals.[1] We designed a questionnaire, in which the first presented the research objective and identification of the interviewee, and the second part included three subsections addressing the place and the status of the child and knowledge about pregnancy and its management, attitudes and practices regarding pregnancy, as well as perceptions of childbirth. We used our network of acquaintances to distribute the questionnaire, such as the physicians we encountered during the annual meetings organized by the Higher Women Consortium as well as those whose contacts were provided by relatives. We equally made use of the phone book which led us to female practitioners, whom we contacted either by phone or by email.[2] We conducted interviews and collected life *in situs* stories with some physicians at their job sites. In a sample of twenty interviewees, fourteen were interviewed either at home or at work, whereas six replied online.

Results and Discussion: Motherhood Identity

Maternity continues to be the "foundation of feminine identity, both at the social and individual level" (Knibiehler 40). In the Cameroonian context, almost no woman is spared by the desire to become a mother:

It is a principle of life. (Physician 10, public hospital).

It [motherhood] really changes our way of seeing things…. A mother plans her life based on her children. They are the ones who give a true meaning to her life. (Physician 9, public hospital).

Such sentiments may be what led Perrot to say that "maternity lasts for a lifetime" (89). When asked whether it is important to be a mother, all the women answered affirmatively. However, one physician said the following: "It is gratifying to be able to give love to a child and to receive love in return. Ideally, every woman would like to be a mother, and this is not always possible. Therefore, this should not be an end in itself" (Physician 2, public hospital). Nonetheless, some people described a mother as "someone of female gender who has given birth or is raising children" (Physician 3, religious hospital). Another physician said: "A mother is first a woman. In addition, a mother has gone through things that a woman would never understand or feel. However, this peculiar aspect does not diminish the fact of being a woman" (Physician 8, private hospital).

Some female physicians clearly distinguish between the woman and the mother. For them, "the woman is a person of female gender while a mother is first a woman and has at heart to contribute to the education and upbringing of a little being"(Physician 5, private hospital). On a daily basis, then, "All mothers are women, but a woman is not necessarily a mother" (Physician 2, public hospital). All women, including mothers, do not possess maternal instinct, as the mother-child relationship is first and foremost a social construct. We can therefore conclude with Knibiehler that maternity "is a matter of women" (35). In fact, whether it concerns the life experience of maternity or social maternity in terms of roles, the motherhood identity expresses itself in many ways (Boni 153).

Being a mother has even changed the medical practice of some female physicians: "The quality of my consultation has changed since I became a mother. There is a real difference between before and now. I am much more careful when I consult or auscultate a child" (Physician 11, religious hospital). From this description, maternity "is a source of identity, the foundation of a recognized difference, even if it is not lived" (Perrot 89). Finally, virtually all women are of the following opinion: "Every woman should have at least one child. She can only give up if it is the will of God" (Physician 6, private hospital). This is probably why physicians do not make a difference between the woman and the mother.

Announcing the Pregnancy, Its Perception and Its Management

The maternity experience is managed everywhere (Jacques). Pregnancy, in contrast represents "a particular and long moment which, by the grace of God, results in a gift of Man (or Men) to humanity" (Physician 1, public hospital). For confirmatory purposes, some women do a pregnancy test, whereas others follow physiological signs:

> To have confirmation of my pregnancy, I did a blood test. In fact, I had already done a pregnancy test which was positive. Although I had nausea and vomiting, I was not certain of the results so I opted for a blood test which confirmed the first results. With my husband, who is not part of the medical corps, being out of the country, I snapped the test strip and sent it to him via WhatsApp [laughs]. He did not understand it at all. Then I told him that I was pregnant [laughs] (Physician 6, private hospital).

> In my case, it is the amenorrhoea and vomiting, which alerted me.... I announced it to my husband during a conversation. (Physician 16, public hospital).

Even though pregnant women may announce their pregnancy to their partner, parents, siblings and friends, they do not all behave the same way once the pregnancy is confirmed. Indeed, for them, pregnancy is first of all a physiological phenomenon.

Consequently, it is seen as a disease. However, because of the risks and complications related to pregnancy, some of them fear it:

> Pregnancy is not a disease. But it scares me because I vomit a lot all throughout my pregnancy. (Physician 16, public hospital).

> Many questions go through my mind. What if things don't go well? When the baby does not move, I panic. There are always fears and many what ifs [laughs] (Physician 6, private hospital).

> Pregnancy is scary because of its risks and possible complications (miscarriage, bleeding during pregnancy, diseases linked to pregnancy). (Physician 1, public hospital).

> Pregnancy scares me because I know the risks and all the possible complications. (Physician 15, public hospital).

> Pregnancy scares me because I have already lost a baby. But outside that, it is a state which should normally not scare me. (Physician 8, private hospital).

> Before I was very scared. Now that I have become mother myself, no more [laughs] (Physician 11, religious hospital).

In view of their obstetrical knowledge, some female physicians who are conscious of the risks are worried about being pregnant. They are in two categories: those who work without letting their pregnancy become an obstacle to exercising their profession and those who do slow down their activities because of their pregnancy.

One physician, and a mother of four, belonged to the first category: "My pregnancies have always been uneventful. I work until the last week" (Physician 3, religious hospital). This is not always the case for some, who despite the absence of fear start their pregnancies with sympathetic signs such as vomiting, nausea: "When I am pregnant, everyone notices it. I am bedridden throughout the first trimester. I vomit endlessly.... During the first two months, I do not feel well. I got scared the first time. After the first trimester, it is cool" (Physician 10, public hospital). For some female physicians, besides the visible hormonal problems (e.g., vomiting and nausea) pregnancy is absolutely not scary. It is the context in which the women live their experiences that makes them anxious: "Because we live in Cameroon and the indicators for maternal and neonatal health are very poor; this is worrisome for a future mother" (Physician 5, private hospital).

> Once I notice that I am pregnant, averagely around eight weeks of amenorrhoea, I start the antenatal visits because I often have difficult pregnancies. That is when I also do the first echography to confirm the pregnancy and verify the number and quality of fetus. (Physician 16, public hospital).

> I start with the consultations as from the first month because there are diseases and anomalies that can be diagnosed early and would determine the outcome of the pregnancy. (Physician 5, private cabinet).

> I go there as soon as I am pregnant because the follow-up is very important for the baby and the mother. (Physician 8, private cabinet).

> I go there as from one month to detect anomalies susceptible of being managed to protect the baby. (Physician 7, public hospital).

Those who consult their obstetrician-gynaecologist (OB-GYN) in the second trimester have a common attitude with many women, who continue to maintain the cultural secrecy of the first trimester of gestation (Ewombè-Moundo 43). They wish to keep their pregnancy a secret for as long as possible. They also mentioned several other reasons, including their medical knowledge and laziness:

> As a physician, I know exactly what to do. I know the problems that can be associated with pregnancy. I therefore go to the hospital when it is necessary. I know what to avoid. (Physician 10, public hospital).

> Personally, I consult after about three to four months of pregnancy if I do not have any major undesirable effect. But prior to that, I have already done an echography, and I am already self-medicating with iron and folic acid. (Physician 2, public hospital).

> I went to consult at three and a half months because I am able to identify the signs of danger... In fact, I don't go there because of negligence [bursts of laughter]. (Physician 6, private cabinet).

We notice that although female physicians postpone their medical appointments, during the antenatal period, they take care of themselves due to their medical knowledge and even perform their own obstetric ultrasound.

> My knowledge of medicine improves my habits and enables me to be stronger when faced with difficulties related to pregnancy. (Physician 4, public hospital).

> I do the obstetric ultrasound to confirm the pregnancy and verify the implantation of the embryo. (Physician 8, private hospital).

> I do it to assure myself that there are no fetal malformations. (Physician 2, public hospital).

The participants also mentioned that the knowledge they possess regarding pregnancy and its outpatient management led them to take care of themselves:

> My first two experiences traumatized me. Therefore during the last pregnancy [her fourth], I was scared because I had elevated blood pressure during the previous [one]. One of the staff [members] told me words I would never forget. To be candid, I followed up by myself. [As a result, for her pregnancy, she has done everything itself] I literally made my own patient book of

medical history when it was time to give birth. [I was] very disappointed by the quality of health services I received during previous antenatal visits. (Physician 3, religious hospital).

The physicians who slow down their activities while pregnant take time to rest and respect the doctor's instructions. With or without sympathetic signs (vomiting, nausea), they are careful with their health while working a little less than usual:

The activities are practically the same, just slowed down a little due to [my] tiredness and sometimes the discomfort. (Physician 1, public hospital).

I limit my mode of high-risk transportation. (Physician 7, public hospital).

I continue my activities normally, taking care of myself and my pregnancy ... by listening to my body. (Physician 4, private hospital).

Ultimately, every experience depends on how the physician feels. They do not necessarily take into consideration the medical indications that would require a consultation as soon as menses stop (Schilte and Anzouy 57). However, their medical knowledge enables them to make wise decisions.

Perceptions and Experiences of Childbirth

Parturition remains the highlight of the pregnancy experience for female physicians:

"Childbirth presents as the 'critical phase' of maternity both for the woman—because it represents a strong physical and psychological experience—and for the medical team. Indeed, if the pregnancy is monitored ... childbirth is presented as an event [involving risk for the mother and the [new-born]" (Jacques 131). The experience of parturition is variable from one physician to the other. The female physicians are not spared from the limit that exists between the healthcare provider (dominant) and the care receiver (dominated) as well as between the pathological (pain) and the natural. The healthcare provider is represented by the person who manages the parturient and the care receiver by the pregnant woman:

Because I was in labour for forty-eight hours without attaining full dilatation. Being of the medical corps, I feared for the baby. I am very scared of childbirth. Many relatives of mine have had complications during childbirth, and a few died from them. Health professionals are not spared. (Physician 12, public hospital).

The female physicians entrust their pregnancies most often to the OB-GYN, whom they judge as being understanding. However, even if the latter are better equipped than midwives, the female physicians find them less patient during childbirth:

The OB-GYN does not have the time to get into details. (Physician 11, religious hospital).

They usually don't have time, and don't consecrate much of it to their patients. [For some physicians,] they have many patients. (Physician 10, public hospital).

Compared to the OB-GYN, the midwife has "a good knowledge of the possibilities of her hands, of the dexterity in her manoeuvres and her massages, and especially, plenty, plenty of patience and devotion" (Laforce 43). This is not always the case with their colleagues, for whom the caesarean section has almost become a normal mode of delivery. As a result, the female physicians argue that these specialists are likely to send parturients, including themselves, to the operating theatre. In contrast, the midwife takes her time: "Through experience, she has an outstanding mastery of delivery, even the difficult ones; [she gives] small tips to support the parturient during labour, which eventually helps her to give birth vaginally" (Physician 5, private hospital).

The physicians have given birth in both public and private hospitals. A few prefer to deliver in public and/or religious health institutions, whereas others prefer private hospitals. Many factors influence these decisions: equipment and facilities (e.g., operating theatre and incubators), trustworthy relationships, as well as the presence of specialists.

One physician gave birth to all her children vaginally and without external intervention. However, though having benefited from a physiological delivery during her third parturition, she still has bad memories:

During my first experience, I was treated by a gynaecologist who knew that I was a physician. She is not the one who finally made me deliver. Having observed the management of pregnancy and childbirth in another African country, I was very irritated by the way the consultations generally took place. Pregnant women are not informed about the pregnancy experience, the why and how of childbirth; they discover it in the delivery room. In my case, I was not satisfied at all by my first two experiences, even though I was being treated by a gynaecologist.... For my first childbirth, a caesarean section was recommended. I did not accept it because not only did I know my body, but [I also knew] the indications for a surgical delivery. Judging from all the parameters presented by the ultrasounds, [I knew] there was no medical reason to consider a c-section. Finally, I even went beyond the indicated pregnancy term before giving birth vaginally to an adorable baby girl in very good health, in a local health centre. The fees for the caesarean section which had been paid were never reimbursed [sighs].... Fortunately, the delivery went well. I think that the conditions of childbirth here disturbed me and led to a higher blood pressure.... While I was pregnant with my fourth child, I met a very competent colleague and brother [Meaning to belong to the same village] who knew about my past history. For the very first time, I was properly treated.... I once more gave birth without any problem: no tear, no episiotomy. I have very good memories of this delivery. (Physician 3, religious hospital).

This testimony shows that had it not been for her prior knowledge in the obstetrical domain,[3] she would have agreed to be operated upon, even though she was capable of having a normal vaginal delivery judging from her pelvis as well as the weight and position of the fetus.

Another physician, though, affirmed that she was satisfied by the quality of service, although she did ask herself whether her profession had influenced the quality of her management.

I gave birth to my first child at CHU (University Teaching Hospital) where I was doing an internship. They performed an emergency caesarean section because the fetus was not well positioned.... Everything went very well. [Hesitates.] But now, I don't know anymore if the quality of service was because I was working there or because I was a physician. (Physician 10, public hospital).

Regarding parturition, some physicians wish to be cared for by other physicians, whereas others wish to give birth in anonymity. The latter are those who give birth away from where they practice, who do not mention their profession upon checking into the hospital, or who do not give birth where they did their antenatal consultations. For instance, two physicians who worked at hospitals with functional operating theatres chose to give birth elsewhere. One delivered via caesarean section in another hospital located twenty-four kilometres from her job site and residence (Physician 11), and the second travelled 150 kilometres from her home in order for a midwife, with whom she had developed a good relationship, to deliver (Physician 4).

> I wanted to deliver with the person who had been treating me. As the date for which the operation was set did not correspond with his work schedule, I preferred to go where he practiced [Djombe]. In addition, the technical platform here [where she worked] did not suit me. It is not complete. There are no incubators or ambulances (Physician 11, religious hospital).

> I did not want to give birth where I worked.... For my second and third deliveries, I went back there to give birth with the same midwife because I was happy with her services. (Physician 4, private hospital).

Concerning the choice of the institutional actor who would handle the delivery, the preference differed from one physician to another. Although all recognize the competence of the midwife, some preferred to be assisted by a male physician, even though many critiqued them for frequently sending parturients to the operating theatre:

> I prefer to be received by a man. He understands the pain of the woman better than the midwife, because he is of the opposite sex. (Physician 4, private hospital).

> I rather prefer men for reasons of feeling. [Hesitations] Hmm, I don't really know how to express this. (Physician 6, private hospital).

In a previous study conducted by Wogaing the nonphysician parturients had also opted for the institutional actor with whom they felt most understood and supported ("Repenser la parturition"). Despite their preference for male institutional actors in practice, the women also subtly acknowledge the knowhow of the midwife when it comes to delivery.

Generally, the female physicians emphasized the professionalism of the delivery personnel, especially the knowhow of the midwife, who is respected as specialist of vaginal delivery: "In the hospital, the midwife is the person who is best placed to advise the pregnant woman and to manage her pregnancy and delivery" (Physician 3, religious hospital). The OB-GYN is called only as last resort. Overall, most do not focus on the gender of the delivery staff. What matters is their expertise: "It does not matter who assists me as long as they are professional" (Physician 8, private hospital).

The experience of most physicians is not different from the life stories of other women (Wogaing, Deliver at Douala – Cameroon: a real challenge). The outcome of childbirth is comparable to that of non-physician women. Among our interviewees, we noted and created different categories concerning the birthing experience: the happy[4] the bruised but happy, the near misses, the c-sectioned, and the damned. Regarding the happy ones, these are parturients who had a normal delivery with no tear nor episiotomy. The new-born is healthy. (e.g., Physician 3, religious hospital).

The bruised but happy ones had a physiological delivery, but their new-borns were sick, "poorly made"[5] or passed away during delivery or in the immediate postpartum. As one physician said, "I gave birth to my first baby without any difficulty. Unfortunately, he passed away a few hours later" (Physician 8, private hospital). As for the near misses (Mayi-Tsonga and al.), they had a difficult vaginal delivery and came close to death during delivery and postpartum. They either had an episiotomy or a vaginal and/or perineal tear:

At term, I unwillingly found myself in a district hospital where I was received by a nurse. While on the way, I realized that the situation was getting complicated.... It was as if the nurse did not know much. However, I did not tell her that I was a physician. I was scared that she would abandon me to my sad fate.... I had what is called an incomplete breech. She was supposed to use the Mauriceau manoeuvre .... She did not seem to know it.... Finally, the fetus tore me at the vagina and perineum [sighs]. (Physician 9, public hospital).

I have always delivered vaginally in a clinic. Unfortunately, I have always sustained tears. (Physician 13, private hospital).

The c-sectioned gave birth via a caesarean section. It is often needed when there are fetal -maternal malformations (e.g., small pelvis and a large fetus, placenta previa, etc.), as was the case with two physicians. This mode of delivery is always determined during the prenatal consultations, and some caesarean sections have been done in emergency settings (c-sectioned in-extremis), in which case the surgery had not been planned. Their new-born can be in good health just as much as his fate can be identical to that of the new-born of the bruised happy one.

I was operated upon twice. The first time was an emergency caesarean section due to the mal position of the fetus. The second was elective, and once more, it was because of a fetal malposition on a scarred uterus. (Physician 10, public hospital).

My previous deliveries had been very painful. It happened by caesarean section each time [silence]. (Physician 7, public hospital).

Finally, the damned are those who pass away in the course of the pregnancy or childbirth. This was the case of Hélène Ngo Kana, a young physician and a mother of two. She died following a complication of her third pregnancy: "The patient died following a severe infection which led to the failure of her vital organs. She was pregnant. Having checked into the clinic ... on the 4th of January 2016, she lost her pregnancy during the hospitalization" (Tchundju). Several explanations were put forth to explain the cause of her death. Yet the principal question is how could a female physician die in such a manner in the hands of her colleagues, cognizant of the Cameroonian setting whereby the patient's personality has often influenced the quality of care received? She nonetheless passed away on 10 January 2016 at Douala General Hospital.

Conclusion

The objective of this chapter was to highlight the maternity experiences of female physicians in Cameroon. We opted for a qualitative study and made use of interviews and life stories to understand how these women's experiences. These women are active actors in their pregnancy and sometimes entrust their gestation and parturition to institutional actors involved in childbirth. On the medical level, they do not always go for antenatal consultations at the recommended periods. However, they do not risk practising their delivery by themselves. They may give birth in strict anonymity with the assistance of a nurse and also at the risk of suffering a medical emergency without presenting herself as a physician, or they may mention their profession in a bid to orientate the institutional actor during the delivery process. In the end, the pregnancy and delivery outcomes are identical to those of ordinary women.

We identified different categories of deliveries: happy ones, bruised happy ones, near misses, c-sectioned, and damned. Maternal mortality spares no one, not even the women in white coats who are more equipped than the rest. It is important to humanize healthcare; OB-GYNs need to listen more keenly to the body of the parturient in the same way as the midwives, who are often more patient. There should be real communication between the healthcare providers, the persons accompanying the patients, and the healthcare receivers—even if they are physicians themselves.

Endnotes

1. The Cameroon health system is comprised of three sectors: traditional medicine, public sector, and private sector. The private sector has two subsectors: for profit (private clinics and hospitals) and non-profit (religious hospitals).

2. Concerning the telephone directory, it usually contains the numbers of physicians registered with the national order of Cameroonian doctors. Our approach was equally used by Aline Cohen when she addressed the question of the feminization of medicine with emphasis on the place of maternity in the organization of the work.

3. In the course of her training, physician 3 of the religious hospital had done a long internship in another African country, where she was able to observe the process of managing pregnancy and childbirth.

4. The term "happy ones" refers to the girl or woman who had a normal pregnancy and gives birth naturally without any external intervention. We created this expression during the analysis of data

phase of our doctorate degree in medical anthropology. The terms "bruised happy ones," "near misses," "c-sectioned," and "damned" are also taken from here.

5. "Poorly made" neonates are those presenting with imperfections or infirmities at birth.

Works Cited

Boni, Tanella. Que vivent les femmes d'Afrique ? Panama, 2008.

Cohen, Aline. Être mère et médecin généraliste : la gestion de la maternité. Étude qualitative par entretiens semi-dirigés auprès de 18 femmes médecins généralistes installées dans la région Rhône-Alpes. Médecine humaine et pathologie. Dumas, 2016, dumas.ccsd.cnrs.fr/dumas-01364080/document. Accessed 28 Mar. 2021.

Ewombé-Moundo, Elisabeth. "La Callipédie ou l'art d'avoir de beaux enfants en Afrique Noire." Grossesse et petite enfance en Afrique Noire et à Madagascar, edited by Suzanne Lallemand, L'Harmattan, 1991, pp. 41-60.

Institut National de la Statistique. Enquête Démographique de la Santé. Institut National de la Statistique, 2012, www.statistics-cameroon.org. Accessed 28 Mar. 2021.

Jacques, Béatrice. Sociologie de l'accouchement. PUF/Le Monde, 2007.

Knibiehler, Yvonne. Histoire des mères et de la maternité en occident. PUF, 2000.

Laforce, Hélène. "L'Accouchement traditionnel d'hier à aujourd'hui." Accoucher autrement, edited by Francine Saillant and Michel O'Neill, Saint Martin, 1987, pp. 40-46.

Mayi-Tsonga Sosthène et al. "Audit de la morbidité obstétricale grave (near miss) au Gabon." Cahiers Santé, vol. 17, no 2, 2007, pp. 111-15.

Perrot, Michelle. Mon histoire des femmes. Seuil, 2006.

Schilte, Christine, and Françoise Auzouy. La Grande aventure de votre grossesse. Hachette, 1991.

Tchundju, Bravo. "Décès du Dr Hélène Ngo Kana : l'ordre des médecins revient à la charge." Camer, 10 Feb. 2016, www.camer.be/49474/11:1/cameroun-deces-du-dr-helene-ngo-kana-lordre-des-medecins-revient-a-la-charge-cameroon.html. Accessed 28 Mar. 2021.

Wogaing, Jeannette. "Repenser la parturition : le genre masculin comme modèle préférentiel au cours de l'accouchement à Douala (Cameroun)."*Revue Aba*, no. 5, 2017, pp. 87-106.

Wogaing, Jeannette. *Maternité et décès maternels à Douala (Cameroun): Approches socio-anthropologiques.* Thèse de doctorat en anthropologie. Strasbourg/Douala. Université de Strasbourg/Université de Douala, 2012.

Wogaing Jeannette. "Deliver at Douala: A Real Challenge." *Missing the Mark? Women and the Millennium Development Goal in Africa and Oceania*, edited by Naomi Mcpherson, Demeter Press, 2016, pp. 212-33.

Notes on Contributors

Rohini Bannerjee (she, her, elle), born and raised in Dartmouth, Nova Scotia, daughter of immigrants from Himachal Pradesh, India, is an associate professor of French in the Department of Modern Languages & Classics, graduate coordinator of the International Development Studies Program and a faculty member in the Asian Studies, and Graduate Women & Gender Studies Program at Saint Mary's University, Halifax, Canada. Rohini's primary research focuses on the literatures and cultures of the Francophone Indian Ocean.

Sally J. Bird is an academic paediatric anesthesiologist She has an interest in procedural sedation, patient safety, regional anaesthesia, and improving the perioperative experience for all children and families. She has been married for fifteen years to a psychiatrist, and together they have three children.

Alekhya "Baba" Das, PhD (he/him) is a Research Associate for the 'Participatory Arts for Seniors' research project (a partnership of Govt of New Brunswick [NB], University of New Brunswick and Art4Life Inc). As a NBHRF Postdoctoral Fellow, Das's prior research examined domestic violence in NB. Das has a doctorate in Sociology from the University of New Brunswick.

Hannah Rochelle Davidson is an undergraduate at Hampshire College in Amherst, MA, USA studying reproductive health. She worked as a full-spectrum doula in the Western Massachusetts region before returning to school to finish her degree. She hopes to complete an MD and a PhD in family medicine and anthropology, respectively.

Arundhati Dhara, MD, MPH is a family doctor practicing in Mi'kma'ki (Nova Scotia). Her clinical appointments include hospitalist work in Dartmouth, NS and primary care on Sipek'nekatik First Nation. She is also a regional physician advisor with Indigenous

Services Canada and a Co-Director of the Medical Humanities Program at Dalhousie University.

Hannah Feiner was born in Fredericton, NB, and grew up in London, Ontario. Her publication credits include *"The Geminis" and "Supine" in Ballyhoo 2001: Plays from London, Ontario* (2003, Ed. Jeff Culbert) and "robin's egg" in Hart House Review (2002, Ed. Jennifer Bronson). Hannah is a family doctor at St Michael's Hospital. She lives in Toronto with her husband and daughters. Hannah is working on a collection of creative nonfiction about living with an astrocytoma.

Kimberly C. Harper is an associate professor of English at North Carolina Agricultural and Technical State University in Greensboro, NC. She is currently researching and writing about diversity in technical communication, the visual narrative of Black maternal heath, and mental health within hip-hop culture.

Ajantha Jayabarathan began medical practice in Nova Scotia in 1991. She worked alongside faculty in the Dalhousie department of family medicine and was the clinical administrator of their teaching sites. She then set up a private practice in Halifax. She has pioneered the transformation of office practice to be managed electronically and successfully piloted the "MyHealthNS" patient portal. Shared mental health care, collaborative healthcare with traditional and complementary practitioners, and healthcare advocacy are of deep interest to her practice. Currently, Dr. Jayabarathan cares for twelve hundred patients, with the help of a dedicated group of likeminded interdisciplinary professionals at the Coral Shared-Care Health Centre (http://coralsharedhealthcare.ca/)

Anna Johnson is a writer, researcher, and mother in East London, UK. She studied history and theory of art (BA Hons., Kent) and has a MA in fine art (Central Saint Martins). Anna is undertaking a creative writing PhD (Kingston), focusing on her experiences of motherhood. Her published writing includes "Objects of a Maternal Haunting" in *Everyday World-making*, 2018. https://annaotheranna.wixsite.com/mysite

Catherine Ma, PhD is an associate professor of psychology at Kingsborough Community College. Dr. Ma earned her doctorate in Social-Personality Psychology from the Graduate Center of the City

University of New York (CUNY) with a certificate in interactive technology and pedagogy. She has presented and written extensively on the maternal experiences of breastfeeding, mothering challenges, and critiquing the current breastfeeding paradigm. Born in Kowloon, Hong Kong, Dr. Ma is a naturalized citizen of the United States and an active board member of the Asian American/Asian Research Institute of CUNY. Her current research focuses on how to counter negative stereotypes of immigrants among community college students and she is a mother to three.

Sharon McCutcheon is a Canadian female family doctor in Sussex, NB. She attended McMaster Medical School while mothering three children. In 2011, she was diagnosed with a brain tumour and returned to work after three surgeries within six months. Dr. McCutcheon is now on permanent disability due to seizures.

Karim Mukhida (he, him) is an assistant professor in the Department of Anesthesiology, Pain Management & Perioperative Medicine at Dalhousie University in Halifax, Canada. He was born and raised in Nova Scotia. In addition to postgraduate medical training at the University of Toronto and Dalhousie University, he has completed a PhD in neurobiology and an MBA. His areas of practice include neuroanesthesia and acute and chronic pain medicine.

Erin Northrup is the mother of four small children. She recently completed a Masters of Applied Health Services Research from the University of New Brunswick. She has an interest in qualitative motherhood research; her thesis focused on the experience of breastfeeding after birth trauma. In her free time, she is a volunteer with a national women's health organization offering mothering support at the local, national and international level.

Celeste E. Orr is teaching faculty at St. Lawrence University. Their work explores the intersection and discursive construction of intersex and disability as well as compulsory dyadism and able-bodiedness.

Ariel Watson is an associate professor of modern and contemporary drama at Saint Mary's University. Her research (published in *Modern Drama, Theatre History Studies, Canadian Theatre Review,* and elsewhere) deals with metatheatre, representations of psychotherapy and mental illness in the theatre, national theatres, and immersive performance.

Her current project grapples with the ethics of spectatorship and the influence of gaming in immersive theatre. She is a citizen of the United States, a permanent resident of Canada, and the mother of Winter (age six).

Amanda D. Watson is teaching faculty at Simon Fraser University. Her work examines gendered and racialized labour responsibility, paid and unpaid carework, and maternal affect.

Darryn Wellstead is a PhD candidate in Sociology at the University of Ottawa. Her dissertation research examines the intersection of mothering, social media, science, and medicine. Darryn is also a faculty member at Northern Lights College in Fort St. John, BC, where she teaches courses in sociology, anthropology, communications, and women & gender studies.

Jeannette Wogaing is senior lecturer in the Department of Anthropology at the University of Douala, Cameroon. Her research interests include traditional and contemporary patterns of motherhood and fatherhood in Cameroon, women in academe and women in prison.